Total Fitness
Training for Life

Total Fitness
Training for Life

Joe Henderson

wcb
Wm. C. Brown Publishers
Dubuque, Iowa

Other Books by the Author

Long, Slow Distance (1969)
Road Racers and Their Training (1970)
Thoughts on the Run (1970)
Run Gently, Run Long (1974)
The Long Run Solution (1976)
Jog, Run, Race (1977)
Run Farther, Run Faster (1979)
The Running Revolution (1980)
Running, A to Z (1983)
Running Your Best Race (1984)
Running for Fitness, for Sport and for Life
    (1985)
Joe Henderson's Running Handbook (1985)

Cover credit © Kaz Mori/The Image Bank
Illustrated by Don Person

Library of Congress Catalog Card Number: 87–72275

ISBN 0–697–00240–3

Printed in the United States of America by Wm. C. Brown Publishers
2460 Kerper Boulevard, Dubuque, IA 52001

10 9 8 7 6 5 4 3 2 1

Dedicated to Uncle Kent King, who first showed me the values of fitness by living them before this was fashionable.

| Contents

FOUR YOURSELF 111

▌*Tables*

Figures

Preface

This book asks you to become more active than you might have been in a long time, or perhaps ever. Before you accept advice that might change dramatically the course of your life, you should first judge the author's qualifications and limitations for outlining that new path.

I readily admit to not being an expert on the highly technical aspects of fitness. I report here the fitness techniques of many authorities, but I myself claim no professional credentials as an exercise physiologist, doctor, or fitness instructor.

My main source of authoritative information is Dr. George Sheehan, whose advice forms the backbone of this book. You'll get to know him and his ideas in the Week 2 chapter, but let me introduce him now with a personal endorsement.

To my mind, no one expert better synthesizes the physiology, psychology, philosophy, and practice of fitness than Dr. Sheehan. As a physician, he knows the physical effects of exercise. As a writer and lecturer, he deals with the emotional aspects. As a competitive runner and triathlete, he puts his expertise to practical use.

I've worked as George's editor for most of his writing career, during which time we've come to think somewhat as one. Originally, we'd planned to co-author this book. Other concerns kept him from playing an equal writing role, but in a real sense the book is still his.

I am here as a reporter and a practitioner of fitness whose experience in both areas is personal and long-term. I've been a runner through all or parts of four decades, and a running writer/editor for almost that long. I've conducted daily experiments in the laboratory of the body and mind and have reported the successful tests of myself and other practical experimenters.

This book may appear slanted toward running. That merely reflects my background. However, most of the lessons from my favorite activity transfer directly to related ones. Wherever you see the word *run*, translate it to read *walk, bike, swim,* or any other type of prolonged movement. Any choice from the aerobic family is the key component for the type of fitness promoted here.

In my teens, I took fitness for granted. It wasn't a goal in itself but an automatic by-product of the way I lived: working on a farm, eating the wholesome products of the farm and garden, living slowly and quietly in a small town, walking or bicycling a paper route, playing a variety of sports.

I was 14 years old and already fit when running became my special sport. I never have run purely for exercise, but was attracted to it first for the excitement of competition and stick with it now as a relaxing recreation.

I would have run 99.9 percent of the last 10,000 days even if it had done me no good physically. Whatever physical fitness it gave was, and is still, a by-product of more immediate rewards of doing what I enjoy.

The running surely does promote fitness. Direct benefits include a well-tuned aerobic system and the luxury of eating my fill without gaining weight.

Running also promotes good health habits indirectly. For instance, I've never smoked and rarely drink alcohol. Concerns over effects on today's performance are more effective in controlling these vices than warnings about their long-term damage.

Having patted my own back, I must now confess that my approach hasn't been the best one for overall fitness. George Sheehan says, "Fitness is a stage you pass through on the way to becoming an athlete." The work of maximizing results is too hard and too specialized to promote balanced fitness.

Athletes are often *less fit* than moderate exercisers in terms of balanced development. I was less fit at my competitive peak than when I started running and than I am now.

In my 20s, I practiced no supplementary exercises and no alternative sports. I paid little attention to diet except as it directly affected performance. I accepted chronic physical fatigue and emotional strain as the prices of success.

I regret none of this, but also know I couldn't have gone on living indefinitely this overspecialized, overstressed way. A more sensible approach has replaced it in my 30s and 40s.

Running-induced injuries forced the adoption of stretching exercises into the daily routine, along with the replacement of some runs with walking, bicycling, or swimming. Unbalanced muscle development, strong legs under an atrophied upper body, led to adding small amounts of strength training.

Several nutrition-related health crises in my family, plus some late-blooming allergies of my own, inspired dietary changes. Running evolved from being a cause to a cure for tiredness and tension.

My history reflects the story of the fitness movement in recent years. The trend is away from overemphasis on a single activity—be it aerobic, muscular, nutritional, or stress-reduction—and toward total fitness.

This book takes a total, well-rounded, long-range approach. I hope to teach you its ingredients and their combinations faster than I learned them, and hope you enjoy your results as much as I have mine.

A special note of appreciation is extended to Professors Anthony Wilcox (Oregon State University), Bob Cross (Salisbury State College), Don Bergey (Wake Forest University), and Don Childs (Alvin Community College) for their very helpful reviews of the manuscript.

Joe Henderson

Study Guide: Teaching Yourself Fitness

Congratulations! You have just taken the longest step toward becoming more fit. By buying this book and perhaps enrolling in a fitness class, you've found dissatisfaction with yourself and made the commitment to change.

The material is presented with several assumptions in mind:

- *You aren't as fit as you want to be.* Either you've never done regular and formal physical training before, or you've failed in earlier attempts and are seeking a better system. You're already sold on the values of exercise, and now are more concerned with how to start training than why you should begin.

- *You don't want to make fitness a second job.* You don't intend to become a competitive athlete or an expert in exercise physiology. You have neither the time, the energy, nor the ambition to spend more than a few hours a week becoming or staying fit. You want the physical activity to be tolerable and practical.

- *You can't depend on group support or access to sophisticated facilities and equipment.* You may have joined an organized fitness program led by a qualified instructor at a well-equipped facility. More likely, however, your fitness activity will be do-it-yourself. You should learn the basic rules of training, take an uncomplicated and inexpensive approach, and be prepared to take responsibility for your own workouts.

These assumptions shape the format of the book. Its material is practical and informal, not theoretical or technical. This is meant to be an activity course in which the descriptions of the activities are secondary to and supportive of the exercise and health acts themselves.

The search for a more perfect you can be made highly technical, as well as expensive and demanding. But it doesn't have to be that way.

This book's program isn't difficult to master. We're not dealing with neurosurgery or nuclear physics, not even with computer programming. Fitness is a simple subject, reduced here to its simplest terms.

What you find outlined here may not be the best of all programs, but it surely is the most basic which still contains all the necessary ingredients. This plan requires no special equipment or facilities that aren't readily available to everyone, no ongoing fees or dues, no teacher or partners, no complex formulas or techniques. It does not require extreme time commitment, effort, or self-sacrifice.

To gain and maintain fitness, you need to adopt good fitness habits *permanently.* They are more likely to last if they become a comfortable and enjoyable part of your normal life than if you are straining to stay fit.

Exercise—especially aerobic activity, most notably brisk walking and gentle running—receives the most attention here (for reasons noted in the Preface and the Week 1 chapter). Aerobic activity is also the simplest and cheapest type to adopt, and it yields the most immediate and dramatic fitness benefits.

The book first introduces you to an exercise program. From there, you move to areas of "life-style" fitness: treating and preventing medical problems, diet and weight control, stress management, and self-improvement. Through it all, the focus remains on the special needs of the active person you have become.

Your total-fitness course takes the following paths:

1. *The Months.* This introductory program is designed to last three months. That allows one season of the year, or about the length of a school term, to acquire new sets of habits.

2. *The Weeks.* Thirteen chapters, meant to be read one each week, cover thirteen topics. The first week covers fitness as a whole. Then you spend three weeks in each of the other major subject areas (exercise, health, diet, and mental training).

3. *The Days.* Each weekly chapter has four sections, each intended to be read on one of the four recommended days of physical training per week. The lessons open with a "Task for the Day" and close with a "Thought for the Day" to preview and summarize the advice.

4. *The Hours.* Exercise periods fit easily into an hour, including time spent getting ready to train and cleaning up afterward. Actual activity time can be as brief as 30 minutes a day, or two hours a week.

5. *The Minutes.* That's all the time you need to read a day's lesson and to record the results of your activity in the log page included with each weekly chapter.

As you work through these lessons, you write your own story of progress. Make it a dramatic one!

Introduction:
Your Fitness

WEEK 1

Fitness Formula

LESSON 1
The Start

Task for the Day: Introduce yourself to regular physical activity, about 30 minutes of sustained, low-intensity (aerobic) exercise to be repeated at least every other day.

This assumes you aren't now exercising in the way and the amount listed above. Exercise is but one of four aspects of fitness to be covered in this book, and aerobic activity (defined and outlined fully in the Week 3 chapter) is only one among many categories of exercise.

We make aerobic training your first lesson for two reasons. First of all, this is an *activity* course, so what better way to start it than by becoming more active? You will devote most of your exercise time and effort to aerobic training, so this lesson shows immediately what you're getting into. (If you're eager to start working for strength and flexibility right away, jump ahead to the Week 4 chapter for an introduction.) Second, exercise often acts as a catalyst for the other areas of total fitness: weight loss; improvements in diet; relief from smoking, alcohol, other drug habits, and stress. You may make these healthy changes even without exercising, but becoming physically active seems to speed them along.

Another assumption is that you have thought before about starting an exercise program, but have kept putting it off until the urge passed. Don't think about it any longer. Do it!

Don't take time to plan carefully what you'll do. Just plan to begin now, and let what happens today happen. Don't go out and buy new shoes or clothes. Don't sign up for an organized program if you aren't already in one.

Don't try an exercise that requires special techniques you haven't mastered. Don't seek out activities that require special equipment or facilities, or a team or partner.

Don't wait until the urge passes again. Start exercising in a low-tech way. The most basic aerobic activities are walking and running, which carry none of the complications listed above. We all know how to move that way, probably already own suitable shoes, clothes adequate for that purpose, and can walk and run alone almost anywhere without paying any fees.

Today, put on the shoes you find most comfortable for traveling a healthy distance on foot. Dress in clothes that allow you freedom of movement. Plan only to keep moving for 30 minutes. Forget distance and just go by the watch, aiming to keep the effort fairly relaxed. This is not a speed test.

Walk for 30 minutes even if you rarely or never do that. Only if you consider yourself quite active and fit should you try to run for the whole 30 minutes.

If you're a regular walker but only occasionally run, and then just for brief periods, follow that same pattern here. Mix some running into what is basically a walking session. For example, the ratio might be a 1-minute run followed by a 5-minute walk.

What you do today establishes a routine (additions and improvements to come in Weeks 2, 3, and 4), that should continue through this introductory course—and ideally throughout your life.

Thought for the Day: Have you adopted a simple, practical, inexpensive, relatively pleasant exercise that you'll want to and be able to practice regularly?

LESSON 2
The Balance

Task for the Day: Introduce yourself to fitness in the most general sense of the word.

Words don't always mean what they seem to say. Take *aerobics,* for instance. When Dr. Kenneth Cooper brought the word into popular usage, it applied to any type of sustained exercise. Yet it has come to imply dancing vigorously to upbeat music.

Say *fitness activity* today, and the first impression that comes to mind is pumping iron or pushing exercise devices at a club. However, fitness has a much broader definition. In its broadest sense, it is the ability to do work.

Health and *fitness* are closely related but not synonymous words. Health is a passive state, an absence of disabling injury or illness. You can be healthy and still not fit. Fitness is active. It means being able to work longer, harder, faster, and more efficiently. You can't become fully fit without first being healthy, but health of body and mind simply takes you to the starting line. The type and amount of physical activity determine where you'll go from there.

In other words, health and exercise both are parts of the fitness whole. Total fitness is the theme of this book, and that word *total* also needs clarification. Total can mean *absolute*, but that definition implies a level of fanaticism we don't want to promote here. For your purposes here, total means *well-balanced*. That balance can be achieved by exercising as little as two hours each week and by modifying certain health habits.

Total fitness depends on four key elements covered by this book in the following order:

1. *Your exercise.* Exercise is activity that you take because you want to, not because you must. Everyone needs some absorbing physical activity that can be the closest an adult comes to child's play.
2. *Your health.* Good health is the foundation of fitness. Good health isn't guaranteed just because you exercise. While physical activity may yield certain types of health tune-ups, it doesn't promise everlasting freedom from injury and illness. Exercise may even *cause* some problems and does nothing to prevent others.
3. *Your diet.* A balanced diet should include enough of the right kinds of food and drink to keep you moving, but not so much that it leaves you sluggish. Exercisers can eat a little more than people who aren't active, and still not gain weight. Yet exercise does not grant a license for gluttony.
4. *Yourself.* Take time to relax; cultivate a sense of calm, humor, and contentment. Make friends with yourself. Heed the survival instincts signaling fatigue, pain, and tension. By working *with* them instead of against them, you can accomplish more work/play with less stress.

Your total fitness depends on the balance of these four elements. We talk about them in this book as if they were separate pegs, but they're really part of a delicate and interconnected system. When the whole system is fit, it moves along with the coordination of a running animal. But let one part go awry, and the system falls out of synch.

Lameness in one of the "legs" seldom stops you cold. It does worse. It eats away at your joy of moving smoothly. Like a three-legged dog, you can exist without any one of these legs. You might even survive if all of them went lame. But the loss of good function anywhere will surely cause you to limp through life.

Thought for the Day: *Are you limping along with one or more of the pegs of your total-fitness support system not working as it should?*

LESSON 3
The Trends

Task for the Day: *See where you fit into the American fitness profile.*

Before judging your own needs, let's look at the fitness level of Americans in general. The news is both distressing and hopeful.

Children and adolescents have never been less fit, according to several studies released in the mid-1980s. This decline occurs at a time when adult fitness activity is rising.

The first survey, commissioned by the Amateur Athletic Union and Nabisco (1984), tested students ages 6 through 17. Sixty-four percent failed to meet standards of an "average, healthy youngster." The failure rate 5 years earlier had been 57 percent. The U.S. Public Health Service (1984) studied 8,800 children in grades five through twelve. This government agency also gave them low marks in fitness, concluding that "American children and adolescents are not developing the exercise and fitness skills that could help maintain their good health as adults. The minimum requirement of vigorous physical activity is generally accepted as 20 minutes at 60 percent of capacity three times a week. Based on self-reports of activity patterns and of exertion in exercise, approximately half of today's youth do not meet these requirements."

The 1985 School Fitness Survey showed similar results for children ages 6 to 17. "Our kids are just not in very good physical condition," concluded the report's authors. "Many parents are in better shape than their kids."

The good news involves adults. After surveying the fitness habits of mature Americans in the mid-1980s, pollster George Gallup commented that "the country's turn toward the active life adds up to the most fundamental change" he had ever studied in this area.

For the first time since Gallup had asked questions on this subject, more than half of the people questioned (54 percent) said they exercised regularly. One-third of those trained 5 or more hours a week.

Between the non-exercising children and their newly vigorous parents fall the college students of the 1980s. This traditionally has been an age for slipping out of shape. "For generations," reported a 1985 *Newsweek* magazine article, "these were people who slept either too much or too little, exercised mainly by trudging to the cigarette machine in the middle of the night, ate pure junk food most of the time, and then lied about it to their mothers."

However, according to a Gallup Poll conducted for *Newsweek,* attitudes toward exercise are changing at the colleges. The number of students who train without a class requirement hanging over them is soaring.

This survey found that 78 percent of the students exercised voluntarily at least once a week. One in every three exercisers chose to run. Running led weight training by a wide margin (34 to 21 percent) as the favored activity, followed by walking (19 percent) and swimming (18 percent). *Newsweek* also noted, "Half of those who don't exercise regularly plan to start working out in the next year."

Your time has come. You want to change your fitness profile. But before learning how to get where you want to go, you must know your starting point. The first step toward finding any solution is identifying the problem.

You pass this fitness course simply by improving. The less fit you are now, the more improvement is guaranteed.

Thought for the Day: On a scale of A–B–C–D–F, how would you grade your level of total fitness today?

LESSON 4
The Test

Task for the Day: Assess your total-fitness status.

In most cases, you don't need a physician to tell you your current fitness status. You don't require sophisticated tests in an exercise physiology lab. A simple self-evaluation will do.

From the list in Table 1.1, what are your most obvious fitness strengths and weaknesses? Be honest with yourself. Look closely at your habits and capabilities, and decide which ones contribute to and detract from your total fitness. Remember that the more out of shape you are now, the more drastic can be your progress. Anyone who progresses in the fitness game is a winner.

Table 1.1
Your Status

Listed here are ten areas of health and fitness over which you have control. Give each a plus (+) for fitness in that area, a zero (0) for a borderline condition, or a minus (−) for unfitness. Record your results at the end of this test.

1. *Injuries/Illnesses.* Pay special attention to injuries and illnesses that restrict fitness activity. If your problem is temporary, wait until it is cured before starting or resuming an exercise. If your condition is chronic, adjust the program to fit your limitations.
   + = no current problem that limits activity
   0 = exercise causes mild discomfort but doesn't aggravate the problem
   − = pain or fatigue restricts the ability to exercise

Table 1.1—Continued

2. *Diet.* Rate the quality of your eating habits. Food types, amounts, and the regularity of meals all have a direct bearing on physical performance capacity.

     + = seldom deviate from healthy dietary practices

     0 = generally eat well but occasionally surrender to the temptations of "junk food"

     − = pay little attention to what is eaten, when and how much

3. *Weight.* "Ideal" is a personal judgment, not one to be found on weight charts. Determine your own desired weight and how far you miss it.

     + = ideal weight for your age, height and frame

     0 = less than 10 pounds from ideal weight

     − = more than 10 pounds from ideal weight

4. *Smoking.* Nothing good can be said for this habit, which can't co-exist with health and fitness. If you smoke, plan to stop. If you don't smoke, don't start.

     + = never smoked and never intend to begin

     0 = stopped smoking or in the process of quitting

     − = currently a smoker

5. *Drinking.* Alcoholic drinks, taken moderately, cause few problems. The goal is to keep the consumption moderate.

     + = drink alcohol in small amounts, if at all

     0 = occasionally drink too much

     − = frequently overindulge in alcoholic drinks

6. *Pulse.* As aerobic fitness improves, the resting pulse rate typically drops. Test the strength and efficiency of your heart by counting its beats when you are relaxed.

     + = less than the average person's reading of 70

     0 = 70 to 80 beats per minute

     − = pulse of more than 80

7. *Aerobic activities.* These require steady, prolonged effort lasting at least 10 minutes and ideally for 30 minutes. The most popular choices are walking, running, bicycling, and swimming.

     + = participate in one or more of these activities at least every other day

     0 = engage irregularly in aerobic exercises

     − = practice no aerobic activity in the amount recommended

8. *"Muscle" activities.* Some of these activities, such as weight training, build strength. Some, such as yoga-type stretching, promote flexibility. A few, such as gymnastics and some forms of dance, combine these two aspects of fitness.

     + = regularly practice strength and flexibility exercises

     0 = participate in these exercises irregularly

     − = do no exercising of this type

Table 1.1—*Continued*

9. *Stress.* Are you a workaholic? Are you easily annoyed and chronically impatient? If so, remember that knowing how and when to call "timeout" is essential to total fitness.
    + = able to relax at the proper times
    0 = frequently agitated and anxious
    − = chronically tense
10. *Rest.* Are you a sleep cheat? Do you often feel drowsy, even at midday? If so, check how long and well you are sleeping.
    + = sleep soundly and awaken refreshed most of the time
    0 = occasionally have trouble falling or staying asleep
    − = often unable to get the sleep required

Injuries/Illnesses:	_____	Pulse:	_____
Diet:	_____	Aerobic activities:	_____
Weight:	_____	Muscle activities:	_____
Smoking:	_____	Stress:	_____
Drinking:	_____	Rest:	_____

Having taken the test, now think about how best to make your daily health habits healthier. Start working on the weak areas, replacing bad habits with good.

Begin by ranking your scores from Table 1.1 in order of importance, from weakest to strongest. Then record this ranking in Table 1.2. Now skip ahead in the book for immediate advice on your most glaring needs. Strive for improvement, not the elusive and discouraging goal of "perfection." Establish new routines that are comfortable to live with, not struggles to maintain.

Here are ways you might ease into healthier styles of living:

1. *Adjusting.* If you suffer from a chronic injury or illness, accept that you have some limitations but don't use them as an excuse for doing nothing physical. If you can't run, walk. If you can't walk, cycle. If you can't cycle, swim. Do the best you can with what you have been given.
2. *Eating.* Modify what you eat instead of trying (and probably failing) to jump immediately and completely into a radically new diet. Reduce the amounts of animal fat, salt, and simple carbohydrates (refined sugar and flour) in your diet. Increase the amounts of vegetables, fruits, and whole grains.
3. *Dieting.* Make weight loss and then maintenance a long-term project, not a crash program. Don't rely on drugs, or "diet" foods and drinks

Table 1.2
Your Needs

Rate your fitness needs from the most needed (marked with a "1") to the least critical ("10"). Then go directly to the most appropriate sections of this book for solutions to the most pressing problems. Weekly chapter numbers and pages are listed here.

Area	Rating	References
Injuries/Illnesses:	_____	Week 6 (pp. 60–65)
Diet:	_____	Week 9 (pp. 91–95)
Weight:	_____	Week 10 (pp. 100–109)
Smoking:	_____	Week 9 (pp. 96–97)
Drinking:	_____	Week 9 (pp. 97–98)
Pulse:	_____	Week 3 (pp. 29–31)
Aerobic activities:	_____	Week 3 (pp. 26–28)
Muscle activities:	_____	Week 4 (pp. 37–44)
Stress:	_____	Week 11 (pp. 113–122)
Rest:	_____	Week 12 (pp. 125–127)

to make you slim. Combine a little less eating (skipping one item per meal, for instance) with a little more exercise (an extra mile on your feet per day) to control calories.

4. *Smoking.* If you chain-smoke, break the chain and smoke only when you absolutely must. If you smoke irregularly, try to stop completely. If you have stopped smoking, congratulate yourself for making this wise investment in your future health and fitness.

5. *Drinking.* Moderate your alcohol use. Drink if you like, at the appropriate times and places, but avoid getting drunk. Choose beer and wine over the harder liquors.

6. *Traveling.* As a first active step toward lowering your pulse rate, incorporate more self-propelled motion into your day. Wean yourself away from overdependence on machines. Take the stairs instead of

the elevator. Walk from a distant place in the parking lot instead of fighting for a space beside the building's door. Bicycle around the neighborhood instead of driving.

7. *Playing.* In addition to participating in formal aerobic training sessions, make your play more active. Leave the golf cart behind and walk the course. Exchange doubles tennis for singles, half-court basketball for full-court. Supplement the stop-and-go action of touch football or the inaction of softball with the continuous motion of soccer.

8. *Working.* In addition to formal strength and flexibility training, put some voluntary physical labor—involving bending, stretching, and lifting—back into your life. Cut and split your own firewood, for example. Do your own gardening and yard work.

9. *Relaxing.* Set aside a period of time each day that is yours alone, a quiet hour during which you call "timeout" and shift down into a slower mental gear. Use this time for your favorite hobby, one you practice by choice and not necessity.

10. *Resting.* Stop cheating yourself out of sleep. Try to get a full night of it, on a regular schedule. If you must cut a night short, find time for a nap the next day. Recharge your energies by doing nothing.

Thought for the day: *What change in your everyday way of living should you make first?*

Now turn to Table 1.3 to log in your training time for the week.

Table 1.3
Week 1 Training Chart

Record your physical training for the week, including only formal sessions, not
incidental daily exercise. List the actual date, aerobic activity, duration in minutes,
and any supplemental "muscle" exercises. A suggested weekly program would
include four aerobic training days, lasting at least 30 minutes, with not more than
two training days in a row or more than two straight rest days.

Day (Date)	Aerobic Exercise	Duration	Other Exercise
Sunday			
Monday			
Tuesday			
Wednesday			
Thursday			
Friday			
Saturday			

Total aerobic training time for the week: _____

Number of aerobic sessions: _____

Average time per session: _____

PART
One

Your
Exercise

WEEK
2

Physical Training

LESSON 5
The Thinker

Task for the Day: *Introduce yourself to Dr. George Sheehan, an eloquent author on total fitness whose ideas appear frequently in the remainder of the book.*

George Sheehan has spent nearly fifty years studying and practicing medicine. Since he wears an "M.D." after his name, readers of his best-selling books and widely read magazine articles may expect him to write like a doctor and may read him only for the medical messages. As a doctor, George Sheehan is a mechanic of the human machine. He knows how its parts work and how to fix them when they break down. Sheehan, the doctor, knows these facts and writes about them well. He can describe heart conditions with the best of cardiologists and foot problems with the best of podiatrists. But in this type of writing, he is only one author in a crowd.

As a philosopher of fitness and sport, however, Sheehan stands alone. He probably would reject the "philosopher" label as too pompous. But it fits when taken to mean one who sees common things in uncommon ways; one who deals more in "whys" than "hows."

Being a doctor is the least of his qualifications for commenting on physical activity. Medical advice is his least important writing. He is at his best when he examines active people's lives instead of simply diagnosing their injuries. This is George Sheehan, the philosopher.

His *Dr. Sheehan on Running* (Anderson/World, 1975) and *Running and Being* (Simon and Schuster, 1978) were unique contributions to the running boom of the 1970s. His philosophies as expressed in *Dr. Sheehan on Fitness* (Simon and Schuster, 1983) are even more relevant to the general fitness boom of the eighties.

While other writers and speakers with his medical credentials might offer complex fitness formulas, Sheehan tries to simplify his advice. For instance, he tells his readers and listeners to be wary of high-tech programs and to trust their own instincts.

"My main message is: 'I'm not going to tell you anything your body doesn't already know. It will tell you if you listen to it.' I don't tell people anything they didn't once know, but have forgotten. Mostly, they've forgotten about play. They've forgotten about their body."

Sheehan deals more in feelings than facts. His fitness philosophy rests on twin cornerstones: (a) listening to your body and heeding its messages; and (b) letting the child within you out to play. Read closely as the doctor explains his approaches to exercise physiology and psychology.

PHYSIOLOGY

"I think the most liberating concept in exercise physiology has been the idea of perceived exertion," says Dr. Sheehan. "The body knows better than any single test what we should do.

"We don't need to put technology between ourselves and our bodies. We can dial ourselves to 'comfortable,' neither too hard nor too easy, and have complete control over what we are doing. What feels right *is* right. We don't have to worry about carrying devices that measure our pulse or taking stress tests."

Sports psychologist Dr. William Morgan from the University of Wisconsin backs Sheehan's view on perceived exertion. Morgan's studies have revealed a 90-percent correlation between apparent effort and laboratory-measured work loads.

"When I train," says Sheehan of his runs and bike rides, "I use perceived exertion automatically. I don't worry about pace, don't even bother to time myself. I use my body's reactions as a guide."

PSYCHOLOGY

Addressing his second theme, enjoyable activity, Sheehan maintains that sports and fitness training need not be grim obligations, required to keep bad things like weight gain and heart disease from occurring. These exercises should be child's play, which adults never need to outgrow.

"People are not inclined to do something just because it is good for them," he says. They also should enjoy doing it and make it play, which Sheehan defines by paraphrasing Mark Twain: something that serves little purpose but has great meaning.

"We are dealing with one of the primary categories of life," writes Sheehan, "one which resists all logical interpretation. Play has a deeper basis than utility. It exists of and for itself. What we need is to conserve those mysterious and elusive elements of play which make it its own reward. What we do must be fun, or else we won't do it."

This statement does not imply that the health benefits growing out of physical activity are unimportant. Sheehan simply thinks the playful approach is *more* important. He says we first must choose activities we enjoy for their own sake. By doing that, we are eager to practice them regularly. Fitness accumulates as an automatic by-product of having fun.

Thought for the Day: *When was the last time you listened closely to the voices inside yourself, and the last time you went outside to play?*

LESSON 6
The Epidemic

Task for the Day: *Learn about the symptoms and treatment of exercise deficiency.*

An epidemic has swept across the land in the last few generations, according to Dr. George Sheehan. Its grip is slowly loosening as the causes and cures become known, but its incidence remains high.

Sheehan outlines the symptoms: "Are you feeling rundown, sluggish, low in energy? Is simply getting to school or work becoming too much for you? Are you exhausted by 3:00 in the afternoon? Do you feel depressed? Have you lost your initiative?

"If your answers are 'yes,' you may be suffering from a life-style disease that, surveys tell us, affects about one-half of Americans. It is called 'exercise deficiency' and undoubtedly is a leading cause of ill health. No household is exempt."

Sheehan calls exercise deficiency (E.D.) a "self-inflicted disease," rising out of something-for-nothing attitudes. "We think we can enjoy the fullness of life without paying for it," he says, "but that is not the way the world works— or the human machine, either."

This problem feeds upon itself. The less work that E.D. sufferers do, the less they are *able* to do. The easier their life, the harder it is for them to take corrective action.

E.D. victims may plead that they're "too old" or "too busy" to do anything about their problem. What they really mean is they can't summon the energy or enthusiasm to make the necessary time, because they feel older than their years.

"Full-blown exercise deficiency states are evident to the most inexperienced observer," writes Sheehan. "Sufferers are manifestly out of shape. For them, repose is the natural state, and any activity is an effort.

"These extreme cases usually fatigue easily and early, and spend most of the day in physical and mental torpor. They are much too tired when they get home at night even to consider taking any physical exercise."

Even relatively young people are tempted to blame their condition on the aging process. Sheehan, who cured himself of E.D. in his 40s and remains athletic in his late 60s, flatly rejects this argument. He claims that slowing down with age is typical but abnormal.

"It *is* average to slow down, to become less productive, to have a lower physical work capacity," he notes. "However, it is not *normal.* Normal is the best you can be. We are never too old to regain fitness, or too young to start preserving it.

"We need to be physically fit whether we are 20 or 35 or even 70. The ebbing of life can occur at any age. It is settling for less than one's best and is the sort of thinking that has resulted in the widespread incidence of exercise deficiency."

So why is this condition allowed to persist? The most common reason offered by the exercise deficient is "I'm too busy; can't spare the time." This plea also scores no points with Dr. Sheehan, who has worked at three jobs (medicine, writing, and speaking) throughout his 50s and 60s while maintaining a full exercise program.

He says the running makes the extra work possible. "Regular physical activity *gives* you additional time—productive hours unavailable by any other means. Physical activity is itself a *cure* for laziness and boredom. It makes habitual the movement the body needs so much.

"Fitness adds life *today.* When we are fit, we can by definition do more work. The day does not end at noon or at five. The day becomes filled with physical, mental, and emotional activity."

Half of Americans suffer from exercise deficiency, but that statistic can be read another way. It implies that the other half now realize the value of regular activity and are taking the cure.

Sheehan delights in the fact that the exercisers are no longer the small minority they were when he went back into training more than twenty years ago. He is certain that the current attraction to fitness is not a fad, but is instead a renewed awareness of a biological and psychological necessity.

"No matter what the advances are in technology," writes Sheehan, "we will always need the vigor, zest, and stamina that go with a well-trained body. There will never be a time when these qualities go out of style."

Thought for the Day: *Do you lack the time and energy to exercise, or lack time and energy because you* don't *exercise?*

LESSON 7
The Choices

Task for the Day: *Having already made the choice to exercise, now choose better ways to do it.*

"If you decide to change your life and go for health and fitness, what is the most important step?" asks Dr. George Sheehan. "Which choice would you make first?" Sheehan would give exercise top priority. He maintains that "exercise was, is, and always will be the single best thing to do for your health. Like charity, exercise covers a multitude of sins.

"Whatever your other habits are, exercise will have beneficial effects. If you continue to smoke or drink or overeat, exercise still gives some positive results. Despite your failures in handling stress and inability to relax, exercise will still make you somewhat fit."

Many of the other health rules involve self-denial—stopping this, reducing that. Exercise takes away nothing. Instead, it fills a void. Sheehan says exercise "is something you *add* into your life, something that should have been there in the first place. And adding it can ease the pressures of adopting those other recommended measures for regaining and maintaining health."

However, fitness programs often fail just as other attempts at changing habits do. These failures can usually be blamed on the program for not fitting the person attempting it. Fitness experts, as deeply steeped in the science of exercise as they necessarily are, sometimes forget that the body they're trying to shape up has a head attached. The body goes only where a willing mind takes it.

Scientific validity is not enough to ask of a fitness routine. It needs to meet psychological as well as physical requirements. Fitness should be a life-long commitment, and you're more likely to spend a lifetime on activities you enjoy than those you find distasteful.

"The millions of people who enter exercise programs will succeed or fail," writes Dr. Sheehan, "inasmuch as they move beyond the details of fitness—beyond tables and charts and schedules—and into the vital, creative area of play. Beyond fitness-as-work, everyone is a child at play.

"Exercise to lose weight. Run to lower your blood pressure. Bicycle to reduce your cholesterol. Swim to increase your cardiac function. Play tennis to help your breathing. Lift weights to clear your brain. These results of working for fitness are all worthwhile, but you may lose interest in pursuing these benefits if the playful element is missing."

Sheehan thinks that "if play is never discovered, in all likelihood the fitness program will fail. Only people with the proverbial gun in their ribs will persist. Only those under doctor's orders—because of a prior heart attack or some disease requiring exercise—will persevere in an activity that they find boring, mindless, and time-consuming."

He adds that "play is quite the opposite. It occupies us totally, and the time passes without our noticing. It is the priceless ingredient of exercise. Here, we find an inward calm and peace. Here, thinking and feeling have a clarity that occurs almost nowhere else. And here, we discover a wholeness, a completion and an integrity that makes us want to celebrate who we are."

George Sheehan is a longtime runner. But he stops short of being a missionary for running. He's an evangelist for exercise, yes, but does not try to convert the masses to his particular way of exercising.

Dr. Sheehan says he was born to run. He inherited the ideal runner's physique (lean and enduring) and personality (a liking for aloneness). Yet he realizes that his activity might not be right for someone carrying a different set of physical and psychological traits. Sheehan recommends matching the program to the person, not forcing an individual into an ill-suited activity he or she finds unpleasant. How do you find the exercise that fits you best? Choose one that matches your body type and mindset, advises Sheehan. Choose one you enjoyed playing as a child, before you thought of it as "fitness work."

> *Thought for the Day: What were your preferred sports and physical activities before you were old enough to care whether they made you fit or not?*

LESSON 8
The Practices

> *Task for the Day: Teach yourself the requirements of an exercise program and how to test for its results.*

Dr. George Sheehan views exercise as a simple and natural act. So he takes a low-tech approach to it, shying away from complex and expensive programs.

"Many people are uneasy beginning a fitness program," writes Dr. Sheehan. "They see fitness as a high-technology industry. Articles, brochures, and advertisements bombard us with the need for specialists and their special equipment. Fitness centers abound with experts who use sophisticated devices to test and monitor their clients.

"Fitness appears to be safe and sure only when we have access to the evaluations and counseling provided by such centers. The ordinary out-of-shape individual is made to feel he or she should not undertake a fitness program without a guide."

It need not be that way. Marking a starting point and monitoring progress require only "a few common household objects," according to Sheehan: "a mirror, a scale, a tape measure, and a watch." His self-testing plan involves four steps:

1. *Mirror.* "Undress and stand nude in front of it. Your reflection tells all. If you look fat, you are fat. You also know where the fat is. If it is on the face and the belly, it will come off readily. If it is on the hips and thighs, it will be the last to go."

2. *Scale.* "It will register fat you cannot see. Match your present weight against the weight you were when you were last active and athletic. Everything you have gained since then is fat."

3. *Tape measure.* "The scale soon assumes less importance. As you become fit, muscle will replace fat. You may even *gain* weight, although it generally remains constant for the first few months. What will change are your measurements. Use the tape measure and establish those measurements. Check the circumference of your calves, thighs, hips, waist, and chest. As you progress in the fitness program, these figures will tell you about fat loss and muscle replacement."

4. *Watch.* "Use this to establish your present level of fitness. This test requires a place where you can run, run/walk, or simply walk a measured distance of 1 to 2 miles for time. The faster you go, the better aerobic condition you are in. As the program progresses, your pulse rate (also checked by the watch) becomes all-important. The resting rate should decrease substantially as your fitness improves."

Sheehan's exercise formula is as simple as his testing: activity lasting about 30 minutes, done at a perceived exertion between "light" and "somewhat hard," taken about every other day. He elaborates on the factors contained in this plan:

■ *What to do?* "Large muscle mass must be involved in the exercise. The majority of the benefits of exercise occur in the muscles. Therefore, the more muscle used during the exercise, the better. The activity can be a personal choice. Walking, running, swimming, cycling, rowing, cross-country skiing, aerobic dancing, and rope skipping all qualify, along with many other exercises and sports."

■ *How much?* "The average workout should last 30 minutes or more. This activity should be continuous, as in running or biking. Training by time eliminates any attention to miles or laps. There is no need to count anything except minutes."

- *How hard?* "Most exercisers want to know how fast they should go. At what speed should the activity be performed? The answer is simple: Listen to your body. Go at the effort which the body says is comfortable. You could also start by using the 'talk test'—the ability to converse with a companion. This will keep you in the correct aerobic range until you relearn the ability to read your own body." (See the ratings of perceived exertion in Table 3.3.)
- *How often?* "The usual recommendation is to exercise at least every other day but not every single day. Recovery days give the body a chance to recoup between training sessions. Rest time is when the training effect actually occurs in the body, when the body adapts to the stresses applied."

There you have it: Dr. George Sheehan's prescription for curing exercise deficiency.

Thought for the Day: *Can you find as little as two hours a week for exercise, or afford not to make the time?*

Now turn to Table 2.1 to log in your training time for the week.

Table 2.1
Week 2 Training Chart

Record your physical training for the week, including only formal sessions, not incidental daily exercise. List the actual date, aerobic activity, duration in minutes, and any supplemental "muscle" exercises. A suggested weekly program would include four aerobic training days, lasting at least 30 minutes, with not more than two training days in a row or more than two straight rest days.

Day (Date)	Aerobic Exercise	Duration	Other Exercise
Sunday			
Monday			
Tuesday			
Wednesday			
Thursday			
Friday			
Saturday			

Total aerobic training time for the week: _____

Number of aerobic sessions: _____

Average time per session: _____

WEEK

3

Aerobic
Exercise

LESSON 9
The Pioneer

Task for the Day: Introduce yourself to Dr. Kenneth Cooper, the pioneering researcher/author of aerobic exercise.

Don't confuse messengers with originators. Shrewd is the person who capitalizes on a fitness fad by releasing a book or videotape as the craze is peaking. Wise is the person who lays the groundwork from which an exercise boom grows. With no insult intended, Jim Fixx and Jane Fonda might be called messengers. In his *Complete Book of Running* (Random House, 1977), Fixx carried the exercise message of the 1970s. Fonda delivered the message of the 1980s in her workout books and videos.

When the definitive history of the fitness boom is written, the two J. F.'s will be credited with saying the right things at the right times. Kenneth H. Cooper, M.D., will be credited with the original thoughts from which most of today's fitness programs sprung.

In the 1960s, Dr. Cooper plucked an obscure word from a physiological text and made it part of fitness language. When he began experimenting with aerobics in the mid-1960s, exercise meant calisthenics or weight-lifting. The accepted adult sports were golf and bowling. Running was only for boxers doing road work and for young, talented, male athletes training for track or other sports.

Dr. Cooper's first great contribution was to make it fashionable for non-athletic adults to be seen moving about in public under their own power, exercising in general and running in particular. Anything done in the name of a stronger heart and a leaner profile became acceptable.

Cooper's research as an Air Force physician had convinced him of the link between regular endurance activity and good health. He in turn convinced the American public of that fact in his first *Aerobics* book (M. Evans and Company, 1968).

In that book, Dr. Cooper presented compelling arguments for aerobic activity: "These exercises demand oxygen without producing an intolerable oxygen debt (such as sprinting does), so that they can be continued for long periods. They activate the training effect and start producing wonderful changes in your body.

"Your lungs begin processing more air and with less effort. Your heart grows stronger, pumping more blood with fewer strokes, the blood supply to your muscles improves, and your total blood volume increases.

"In short, you are improving your body's capacity to bring in oxygen and deliver it to the tissue cells, where it is combined with foodstuffs to produce energy. You are increasing your oxygen consumption and, consequently, your endurance capacity."

He spoke just as convincingly of a more immediate and visible benefit: the effectiveness of endurance work in weight reduction. Each mile of running or walking, or equal effort in other activities, consumes about 100 calories.

The first and most lasting evidence of Cooper's influence was an explosion in the number of runners. He didn't specifically write a running book. *Aerobics* was an exercise text, listing running as one option among many. He didn't mention the word "jogging." Still, the message was clear: Cooper favored running as a fitness activity.

"The best exercises are running, swimming, cycling, walking, stationary running, handball, basketball, and squash—and in just about that order," he wrote. He now lists cross-country skiing at the top.

The body requires continuous activity and isn't too particular about the type. But running is a quick (walking takes longer) and practical (biking and swimming require special equipment or facilities) way to reach the quota of aerobic exercise that Cooper recommended. His quota has both lower *and* upper limits.

In the late 1960s, Cooper presented the radical message that people should exercise more; they were suffering from inactivity. Looking back twenty years later on the running boom that he helped inspire, he observed that runners might be healthier and fitter if they trained *less.*

Cooper and his staff at the Aerobics Center were "overwhelmed" by the incidence of injuries in people running more than 25 miles a week. While a competitor might gamble on higher mileage for greater rewards, this effort is self-defeating for an exerciser whose main goal is to stay active. For non-racers, Cooper sets minimums and maximums: no less than 2 miles, three times a week, and no more than 3 miles on five days.

Converting those distances to the time standards we use in this book, we're talking about someone who runs at 10 minutes per mile—a typical pace for beginners—running 20 to 30 minutes. Hence, our general recommendation of a 30-minute exercise period for runners and equivalent times in other activities. We split the difference between his three- to five-day program and recommend four training days a week.

Thought for the Day: Are you currently exercising at least Dr. Kenneth Cooper's minimums of 2 running miles in about 20 minutes—or its aerobic equivalent (see Table 3.1)—three days a week?

LESSON 10
The Activities

Task for the Day: Find supplemental or substitute paths to aerobic fitness besides running.

Can you spare four hours a week for physical training? That's all the time you're asked to invest in this book's exercise programs, and as little as half of that time need be spent actually exercising.

Gaining and maintaining physical fitness takes time and effort, but not as much of either as you might have thought was required. Exercise of moderate amount and intensity, taken regularly, yields greater long-term benefits than sporadic bursts of hyperactivity.

The programs in this book emphasize moderation and consistency. Advice is framed in terms of minimal requirements, not the most work you can tolerate. You're welcome to put in more than the recommended time and effort. But if basic fitness is your only goal, you don't *need* to do more. Exceeding these recommendations may, in fact, detract from the goal by making the exercise too difficult or impractical to tolerate in the long term.

How much is enough? Thirty minutes of continuous, low-intensity activity—supplemented by a few minutes of flexibility and strength exercises—four days a week. Aerobic training obviously demands most of the time you spend exercising, since by definition it must be continued for extended periods to do much good.

Dr. Kenneth Cooper has identified the best aerobic activities as "running, swimming, cycling, walking. . . ." To this list, first published in the 1960s, add the newly popular cross-country skiing, rowing, and aerobic dancing. Anything that keeps you moving steadily is beneficial.

You're free to choose any of the activities or, better yet, mix them during a week or from season to season. The body merely demands some type of aerobic activity, and the mind thrives on variety. For practical reasons, however, your staples probably will remain walking and running. (Table 3.1 lists the ways to approximate the aerobic benefits of walk or run with other exercises.)

Table 3.1
Your Options

Dr. Kenneth Cooper, the aerobics pioneer, prescribes for fitness runners a workout of 2 to 3 miles. At 10 minutes per mile, this involves a 20- to 30-minute exercise period.

Running isn't a requirement, however. You can substitute or supplement with other aerobic exercises. This table lists their rough equivalents in terms of efforts and benefits, as adapted from Cooper's recommendations:

1. Bicycling, swimming, and cross-country skiing match running minute for minute in terms of efficiency, provided effort levels are comparable.
2. Walking takes about twice as much time to achieve benefits similar to running.
3. Stationary exercise machines can simulate biking, cross-country skiing, and rowing. Running can be done in place or on a treadmill.
4. Active games include soccer, basketball, handball, and racquetball, with only the time spent in motion counting toward the total.
5. These are daily amounts. Plan to train four days each week.

Activity	Time Periods
Running (2–3 miles)	20 to 30 minutes
Bicycling (6–8 miles)	20 to 30 minutes
Swimming (900–1200 yards)	20 to 30 minutes
Cross-country skiing (2–3 miles)	20 to 30 minutes
Running/walking (2–3 miles)	30 to 45 minutes
Aerobic dancing	30 to 45 minutes
Rowing	30 to 45 minutes
Walking (2–3 miles)	40 to 60 minutes
Active games	40 to 60 minutes

While emphasizing endurance training, don't ignore two other aspects of physical fitness: flexibility and strength. Aerobic training helps little in these areas, and may actually have negative effects.

Running, for instance, may lead to unbalanced and overly tight muscle development. The legs train, while the upper body goes along for the ride. The backs of the legs grow strong and tight, while the muscles in the front don't develop to the same extent and strength imbalances result.

A few minutes spent on basic strength and flexibility exercises will maintain proper balance and range of motion. (These are introduced in Week 4.)

Thought for the Day: How, if at all, do you want to mix other aerobic activities into the basic walk/run program?

LESSON 11
The Schedule

Task for the Day: Learn more about the three key elements of an aerobic training plan.

As you set up a schedule, keep in mind the word *FIT.* Its letters can be made to stand for the three critical elements of any program: Frequency, Intensity, and Time. Put another way, you need to know how often to exercise, how hard, and for how long.

Combine the following advice to form your own general training plan in Table 3.2. These recommendations are based on the combined advice of Dr. George Sheehan, outlined in Week 2, and Dr. Kenneth Cooper.

FREQUENCY

Four days of training a week, with no more than two training days in a row and no more than two straight days off between workouts is recommended.

Why this often? Because you need both regularity and recovery time to benefit from the activity. Train too seldom, and your program lacks continuity. Train too often, and you risk chronic fatigue (both physical and mental).

If weekends are your easiest place to find free time, schedule training on Saturday and Sunday. Then plan to spread two more sessions through the week: on Tuesday and Thursday, for instance.

If your weekends are crowded, fit all of your workouts into the weekdays. As an example, train Monday, Tuesday, Thursday, and Friday.

Either way, you never exercise more than two days in a row. You don't go more than two days without exercising.

INTENSITY

Exercise hard enough but not too hard. You don't gain and maintain physical fitness without putting in some effort, but excessive effort is wasted.

Contrary to what some fitness "authorities" would have you believe, pain does not equal gain. It merely adds up to more and more pain, until you no longer can or want to exercise.

Table 3.2
Your Week

Write your ideal program. First, choose the physical activity (or activities) you prefer to practice. Then schedule the training for one hour a day (including time for "muscle" exercise and changing clothes), four days a week at the most convenient times. Plan to train no more than two days in a row and to schedule no more than two straight rest days.

Day of Week	Time of Day	Activity
Sunday		
Monday		
Tuesday		
Wednesday		
Thursday		
Friday		
Saturday		

Train, don't strain. Push your limits, but don't struggle past them. Find your own perceived exertion borderline between "comfortable" and "somewhat hard," and stay just below it (see Table 3.3).

If you want a more precise measurement, check your pulse immediately after stopping the exercise. Maximum aerobic pace corresponds to approximately 75 percent of your maximum pulse rate.

Table 3.3
Your Pace

Gunnar Borg devised a scale of perceived exertion that can be used to measure effort in aerobic activity. The numbers roughly correspond to pulse rates (minus the zeroes) at various levels of exertion for young people. Middle-aged and elderly exercisers normally perceive similar efforts at lower pulse because their maximum rate declines with age.

Rating	Perception of Effort	Approximate Pulse
7 and less	Very, very light	70 and below
8 and 9	Very light	80 to 90
10 and 11	Fairly light	100 to 110
12	Comfortable	120
13 and 14	Somewhat hard	130 to 140
15 and 16	Hard	150 to 160
17 and 18	Very hard	170 to 180
19 and up	Very, very hard	190 plus

This top figure is rather difficult to determine without sophisticated testing equipment, so Dr. Samuel Fox (former president of the American College of Cardiology) devised a rule of thumb. Simply subtract age from 170, meaning that a 20-year-old should treat 150 as his or her peak exercising pulse rate.

TIME

Exercise about 30 minutes each training day.* Fit the exercise loosely into a full hour, broken down roughly this way: 5 to 10 minutes of getting ready to exercise, 30 minutes of aerobic activity, 5 minutes for flexibility and strength work, and 15 to 20 minutes for cleaning up.

Why an hour? Because it is long enough to hold an adequate training session, and long enough so you aren't tempted to work too fast. Yet one hour is still short enough to fit into most people's daily routine without straining them for time.

---

*Some aerobic exercises require somewhat more time, in which case you might spend less changing clothes. For example, you can walk without requiring special clothing or a shower.

During aerobic training, forget about how far you run, walk, swim, cycle, or whatever. Think only about how much time you spend exercising. Count minutes, not miles.

This approach offers several benefits. The practical advantage is freedom from designing or measuring routes or counting laps. The bigger reward from time training is more subtle, as switching to the time standard relieves the pressure of racing against time.

The natural tendency when going a set distance is to finish it as quickly as possible, which often means pushing yourself too hard. However, you can't make a period of time pass any faster. In fact, it *seems* to take longer when you try to rush it. So the tendency is to fill the time period at a comfortable pace.

Thought for the Day: *How does the fitness activity you have been following match the F-I-T recommendations here?*

LESSON 12
The Logistics

Task for the Day: *Decide when and where to exercise.*

WHEN?

"But I'm too busy. I don't have time to exercise." Everyone is busy enough to fall back on that excuse. No one has the time if he or she doesn't want to *make* the time. If you want to train, you *find* the time and stick to that time.

No one can give you that time except yourself. Carve a chunk out of your day. Get up earlier, train at noon instead of lingering over lunch, or skip a television show in the evening.

Morning, noon or night, the effects are about the same. When you exercise depends on the time of day when you operate best and when it's easiest for you to make time available.

Some exercisers prefer the first-thing-each-morning routine. It offers several advantages: Seldom is that time pre-empted by other demands; you wake up quicker by literally getting your day off to a flying start; traffic on the streets may be lightest, and the air coolest and cleanest then. The morning also has its down side: The temptation to sleep through this time after a late night is great; you're sorest and stiffest at this hour, and possibly most prone to injuries; it's dark and cold then during much of the year.

Those who train in the evening or at night prefer it for these reasons: They feel loosest and most awake then; it relieves the day's tensions; they like to exercise with other people, and it's easiest to find partners then. The minuses of exercising late: Work, family and social obligations are most likely to eat into that time; winter nights grow dark and cold early; it's hard to delay dinner when you come home hungry and still have a training session ahead.

Noontime exercise is growing in popularity because it avoids some of the negatives of both morning and evening: no darkness, no sleepiness or stiffness, nothing else to do then except eat.

People operating on a set schedule, with an hour off for lunch, may find the time better spent training than eating. The vigorous exercise temporarily blunts the appetite, gives a physical break from mental fatigue, and keeps them alert all afternoon.

The problems with noontime training include finding a convenient place to exercise near the office or school; finding a place to change clothes and to shower at that time of day; feeling rushed to finish exercising within a fixed time period.

Choose the time with the most pluses and least minuses for you.

WHERE?

"But I don't have any place to train." That's the second most common complaint from beginners.

Look around you. "Running country is everywhere," says former Olympic track coach Bill Bowerman. The same could be said for walking. "Open the door, and you're in business. Run right out the door, run in a school yard, on a city street, at the beach, on a country road, or in a vacant lot. Run down a bicycle path, on a school track, around a golf course, through a park, in your backyard, in a gymnasium, in a supermarket parking lot. Anywhere."

Any safe place is suitable for this activity. But some places are better than others. If you have a choice, look for walking/running areas that meet as many of the following criteria as possible:

1. Convenient enough that you don't have to drive to the start and back after finishing most sessions. That can eat up much of your training time. (But don't become so wedded to the home courses that you avoid exploring other territory on days when there is free time to travel there.)
2. Relatively free of auto and pedestrian traffic. This cuts down on risk, air pollution, and self-consciousness.
3. Controlled dog population. Nothing ruins a walk/run faster than an unleashed dog nipping at your heels.
4. Protection from wind and sun. Large trees along any route are a plus.
5. Pleasant sights and sounds. Nice views and silence don't add to the physical benefits of training, but they do make you want to keep coming back for more.

Choose a variety of routes for a variety of reasons and seasons.

Thought for the Day: When can you best find an hour in your day for exercising, and where are the best places to use that time?

Now turn to Table 3.4 to log in your training time for the week.

Table 3.4
Week 3 Training Chart

Record your physical training for the week, including only formal sessions, not incidental daily exercise. List the actual date, aerobic activity, duration in minutes, and any supplemental "muscle" exercises. A suggested weekly program would include four aerobic training days, lasting at least 30 minutes, with not more than two training days in a row or more than two straight rest days.

Day (Date)	Aerobic Exercise	Duration	Other Exercise
Sunday			
Monday			
Tuesday			
Wednesday			
Thursday			
Friday			
Saturday			

Total aerobic training time for the week: _____

Number of aerobic sessions: _____

Average time per session: _____

WEEK 4

Muscle Exercise

LESSON 13
The Needs

Task for the Day: Introduce yourself to flexibility and strength exercises that counteract the tightness and imbalance left by aerobic training.

Ironically, some of the most highly conditioned endurance athletes are less likely than non-athletes to pass simple tests for strength and flexibility—such as lifting a large portion of body weight, doing a number of sit-ups, or simply bending over and touching the fingertips to the floor without bending the knees.

You're asked this week to test your flexibility and strength, then told how to correct deficiencies in following days. Meanwhile, let's establish a case for employing these supplemental exercises.

"When a runner goes into training," says Dr. George Sheehan, a well-known fitness advisor, "three things can happen to the muscles. Two of them are bad." The good one is that you become a better runner.

But if you don't take any exercise except this, then bad things happen. Dr. Sheehan identifies them as "(a) shortening of the strengthened muscles with loss of flexibility, and (b) strength imbalances developing in the relatively unused, neglected muscles."

Many of the popular aerobic exercises have the same negative effects. These don't appear all at once. You may not experience either of the muscle problems during this introductory course. However, the effects are cumulative, and runners/walkers can become increasingly tight and out of muscular balance unless corrective action is taken.

Aerobic activity, by itself, doesn't yield balanced fitness. Some leg muscles grow super-strong as well as tight. Opposing ones grow lazy. Others such as arm, shoulder, chest, back, and abdominal muscles don't get much of a workout as you run/walk.

Lack of flexibility is a notable problem for longtime runners. Extreme tightness exposes them to muscle and tendon injuries that might not occur if they remain supple.

A great advance in recent years has been the growing popularity of so-called "static" stretching exercises. These involve moving slowly to a position at the point just short of discomfort, then holding that position for several seconds.

These stretches differ from traditional calisthenics both in style and effect. The movements in calisthenics are often violent, and can actually exaggerate the tightening they are supposed to prevent. Static stretching gently loosens the muscles.

These are not, as commonly supposed and practiced, most effective for warming up before aerobic activity. You can warm up just as well by starting the particular activity very slowly and then gradually increasing its pace.

Stretching works best to counteract the tightening effects of the run/walk. Therefore, it is best practiced *after* that session. The muscles respond best to stretching when they are warm, not cold.

Running/walking produces specialized strength, affecting mostly the leg muscles. Its effects on the upper body are nil. So if you don't want to turn flabby from the waist up, you need to adopt the strength-building habit.

Exercises as simple as push-ups and bent-leg sit-ups can restore and maintain much of the upper-body strength lost through specialization and neglect. Daily sets of these exercises, in whatever number you can tolerate, will keep you respectably strong.

If you want more advanced development, move into sophisticated forms of gymnastics and weight training. These are beyond the scope of this book, which treats "muscle" activities as a quick, balancing supplement to aerobic activity.

As with the aerobic programs, the muscle exercise routine prescribed here (see Lesson 16) remains low-tech. It employs no fancy equipment or complex techniques, and can be practiced in as little as 5 minutes daily.

Thought for the Day: *Can you add 5 minutes to your exercise time in the interest of muscle balance?*

LESSON 14
The Stretching

Task for the Day: *Consider the basic requirements and techniques for regaining and maintaining flexibility.*

Put this book aside, stand up—knees straight, feet together—and bend forward slowly and carefully. Reach down with your fingertips until the tightening muscles in the backs of your legs won't allow you to go any farther.

Longtime runners, who have ignored flexibility exercises, get hung up somewhere between the knee and the ankle on this test. Their legs are overly tight.

Dr. Steven Subotnick, a podiatrist with a large athletic clientele, says the trait is almost universal among his patients. He estimates that nine in ten of them can't pass this minimum test for flexibility, and that this is a main reason why many of them visit him as patients.

"The runner must be aware of the fact that endurance exercises reduce flexibility," says Dr. Subotnick. "Distance running results in overdeveloping of the muscles at the back of the lower leg and thigh." Tightness results, and chronically tight muscles don't work as they should.

Robert Bahr, former editor of *Fitness for Living* magazine, writes, "The need for flexibility has long been recognized by fitness experts. In both our high schools and the armed services, token recognition of this need is given in terms of calisthenics programs. But evidence now indicates that calisthenics are not advisable for this purpose."

Much of that evidence grew from the work of Dr. Herbert de Vries, author of *Physiology of Exercise for Physical Education and Athletics* (William C. Brown Co., 1986). He separates stretching exercises into two categories: "ballistic" and "static."

Ballistic exercises are the standard, vigorous calisthenics. They feature quick, repeated movements. Static exercises involve slow and rhythmic stretching, stopping and holding a position at the point of first discomfort.

Dr. de Vries strongly recommends static stretching because of its "three distinct advantages":

1. There is less danger of going beyond the safe limit of stretching when the exerciser moves into position slowly and stops before the point of pain. With ballistic exercises, there is a risk of bouncing past the limit and realizing it too late.
2. Energy costs are lower with static stretching, so the exercises don't tire a person for other activities.
3. Ballistic exercises may cause muscle soreness. Static stretching tends to relieve such soreness.

The natural reaction to extra exercise that is fatiguing is to avoid it, thereby taking no stretching at all. The natural tendency when doing bouncing type calisthenics is to bounce too vigorously, thereby defeating the purpose of the exercise.

De Vries says that when a muscle is jerked into extension, it responds by jerking back and shortening itself again. If this jerking back and forth is too violent, soreness results.

When de Vries was working out his static stretching plan, he took a clue from swimmers, who are particularly prone to calf cramping. "Competitive swimmers and swimming coaches know," he writes, "that swimmer's cramp is promptly relieved by gently forcing the cramped muscle into the longest possible state and holding it there for a moment. It was hypothesized that the simple stretching technique that relieves a swimmer's cramp in the calf muscle should also be effective in providing prevention and relief for any muscle that can be put to a stretch."

De Vries advises all exercisers to determine which muscle or muscles are tight and sore, find the muscular attachments of the involved muscle or muscles, and then "devise a simple position in which the attachments are held as far apart as possible with the least possible effort."

He adds that "many yoga exercises have been found useful, since they use the same principles." More precisely, the static stretching exercises are effective because they are based on yoga principles that originated some 4,000 years ago.

One modern proponent of yoga, author Richard Hittleman, sums up the practice this way: "The movements are performed in relaxing slow motion with very few repetitions. No strain should ever be felt. The practice sessions should leave you feeling elevated and revitalized, not drained."

Thought for the Day: Would you rather feel strained or relaxed at the end of an exercise session?

LESSON 15
The Strengthening

Task for the Day: Consider the basic requirements and techniques for regaining and maintaining upper body strength.

Weight training is great strengthening work if you have the time, equipment, and need for it. Lifting free weights or working on weight machines is the surest way, proponents would say the *only* way, to develop maximum strength.

However, rehabilitating neglected muscle strength and then holding it at a minimum acceptable level doesn't require that you buy a weight set or join a health club. As an aerobic exerciser seeking only to balance your program, you can get all the strength work needed simply from moving your own body weight.

Running/walking is itself a form of strength training, since it requires lifting your weight off the ground about 1,500 times per mile. This activity develops great leg strength, but little elsewhere. If you want even more power and spring in your stride, modify the run/walk sessions somewhat. Climb hills or stairs. Possibly add a small number of short sprints. These diversions build strength faster than low-intensity efforts do.

Bicycling delivers benefits of about the same type and degree as running/walking and has similar limitations. Rowing sports train the upper body more than the legs. Other aerobic activities deliver more balance as a natural by-product. Swimming and cross-country skiing, for instance, work the whole body.

One way to get a full-body workout would be to practice one or more of the water or snow sports. Another would be to add enough manual labor to your day that you don't need extra exercises.

However, most exercisers adopt running/walking as their basic activity, and the heaviest object they have to lift each day is a pencil. If you fit this description, you probably need supplementary strength training.

The exercises recommended here follow the book's low-tech, low-cost, low-key theme. None requires much equipment, technique, or time.

All of these exercises use the body weight as resistance. You "lift" it to the limits of perceived exertion, as in aerobic training—finding your own zone between hard enough and too hard.

The advantages over conventional weight training are that you don't need to worry about proper amounts of weight or about dropping a barbell on your foot. The exercises listed here are safe and self-adjusting to your current abilities. Do only the number of repetitions your current strength allows.

- *Sit-ups.* These sit-ups are modified to maximize effects on the abdominal muscles and minimize strain on the back (see Figure 4.1). Sitting up from a bent-legged position accomplishes both aims. It isolates the midsection muscles and eliminates help from the hips and upper legs. You don't need to sit up all the way, since the muscles benefit the most from the initial lift-off.
- *Push-ups.* Do them the standard way, to promote arm, shoulder, and back muscle strength (see Figure 4.2).

Two alternatives to sit-ups and push-ups combine the strength-building effects of these exercises. These substitutes are designed for people who can't or won't flop onto the floor or ground.

Using one sturdy straight-backed chair, place your hands on either side of the seat and lift your full weight off the chair while staying in the "seated" position. Using two back-to-back chairs (about 2 feet apart), place one hand on the top of each. Perform "dips" for the arms and leg lifts for the abdominals.

You can do any or all of these exercises anytime, anywhere—as part of a formal training session or apart from it.

Thought for the Day: How many sit-ups and push-ups can you do?

LESSON 16
The Routine

Task for the Day: Combine the flexibility and strength exercises into a convenient set.

Five minutes a day will keep you as strong, loose and balanced as a runner/walker needs to be. This assumes you want only a quick muscular tune-up and are not training now for ballet or body building.

The six stretching and strengthening exercises in the accompanying illustrations (see Figures 4.1 to 4.6) have been chosen with both benefits and practicalities in mind. You can perform them all within a 5-minute period, right after finishing an aerobic session.

Do the strength work first, then the flexibility—working from lying down to standing up. All but the most severe cases of inflexibility and weakness are reversible with simple corrective exercises.

Whether you choose to practice these stretching or strengthening exercises or not, listen to advice from one authority in this field. His words fit all types of physical activity.

Ian Jackson might be called the "Kenneth Cooper of Stretching." Jackson's *Yoga and the Athlete* (World Publications, 1978) was every bit as revolutionary a book, despite its much smaller sales, as Dr. Cooper's first *Aerobics* text.

Cooper wrote that the way to train most effectively is to run or swim or bicycle steadily and gently, not briefly and violently. Jackson gave similar advice about stretching exercises.

His yoga book was packaged and promoted as how-to information. It describes one man's journey away from the whip-into-shape mentality that dominates athletics to the friendlier methods of the Eastern activity. Jackson emphasized a key phrase in yoga: "Play the edge." This concept makes yoga as different from traditional calisthenics as jogging is from intensive interval training.

Jackson said the vigorous stretching of calisthenics tries to crash through "pain barriers," while yoga nudges them until they move quietly out of the way.

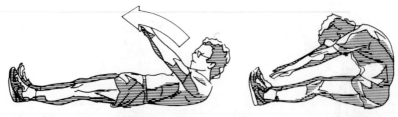

Wrong
Straight-legged sit-ups put strain on
the lower back without giving
maximum development of
abdominal muscles. Legs and arms
do most of the work.

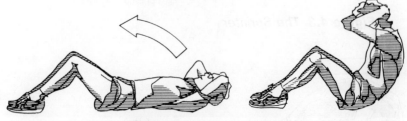

Right
Bent-legged sit-ups relieve back
strain. With hands laced behind the
head (or across the chest) and
knees bent, the abdominal muscles
do most of the work. Most of the
benefit is in the first one foot of the
sit-up.

Figure 4.1 *Safe Sit-ups*

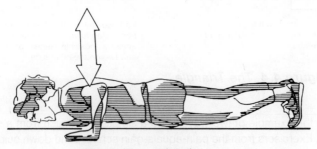

From straight-armed starting
position, touch nose, chest, and
upper legs to floor, keeping back
straight. Work up to twenty or more
repetitions.

Figure 4.2 *Push-ups*

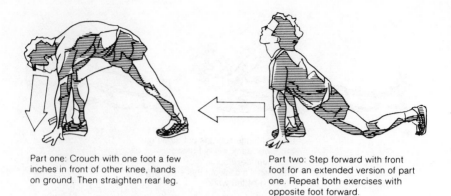

Part one: Crouch with one foot a few inches in front of other knee, hands on ground. Then straighten rear leg.

Part two: Step forward with front foot for an extended version of part one. Repeat both exercises with opposite foot forward.

Figure 4.3 *The Sprinter*

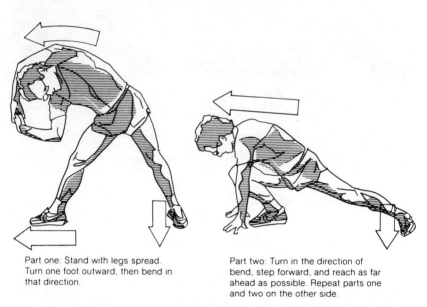

Part one: Stand with legs spread. Turn one foot outward, then bend in that direction.

Part two: Turn in the direction of bend, step forward, and reach as far ahead as possible. Repeat parts one and two on the other side.

Figure 4.4 *The Triangle*

He gave the example of two ways to do a simple floor-touch from a standing position. Exercisers from the pain-equals-gain school bend down quickly. Momentum carries the fingertips to the floor, then a reflex action yanks them up again.

Has this exercise done any good? Researchers such as Dr. Herbert de Vries (see Lesson 14) think not. They say the muscles rebel against this treatment. Their reaction tightens rather than loosens. This sudden movement may even *cause* injury.

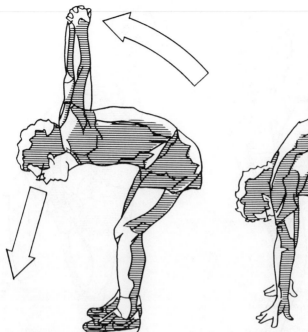
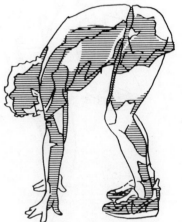

Part one: Clasp hands behind back, stand with feet together and knees slightly flexed. Bend forward while pulling arms upward. Stop at point of discomfort and hold.

Part two: Drop arms until palms touch ground in front of feet. The less flexible you are, the farther in front of the toes you will touch.

Figure 4.5 *The Floor-touch*

The yoga approach is to stretch carefully to the "edge" of discomfort, back off slightly, then hold at that point for several seconds. The first thing you notice is that during the "hold" you ease farther down without really trying. You notice after a few weeks of stretching this way that the edge has moved to a point you could reach only with great pain earlier. You now stretch to it comfortably.

"Playing the edge" means finding that invisible, ever-shifting line between comfort and discomfort. If you never nudge it, you never move it farther out. If you push it too hard, it breaks you. Whatever your exercise is, this rule applies. It works for aerobic and strength training as well as stretching.

Make friends with yourself. Coax out the benefits of exercise instead of trying to drag them out. Listen to the body's messages rather than trying to blot out its screams.

Thought for the Day: *Have you found the winning edge in all of your exercises?*

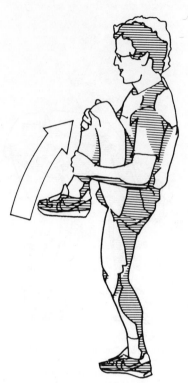
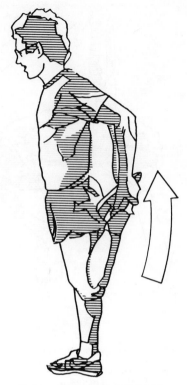

Part one: Cradle a lower leg and pull it toward chest.

Part two: Grasp a foot behind back, and pull toward buttocks. Repeat parts one and two with other leg.

Figure 4.6 _The Leg-puller_

Now turn to Table 4.1 to log in your training time for the week.

Table 4.1
Week 4 Training Chart

Record your physical training for the week, including only formal sessions, not incidental daily exercise. List the actual date, aerobic activity, duration in minutes, and any supplemental "muscle" exercises. A suggested weekly program would include four aerobic training days, lasting at least 30 minutes, with not more than two training days in a row or more than two straight rest days.

Day (Date)	Aerobic Exercise	Duration	Other Exercise
Sunday			
Monday			
Tuesday			
Wednesday			
Thursday			
Friday			
Saturday			

Total aerobic training time for the week: _____

Number of aerobic sessions: _____

Average time per session: _____

PART
Two

Your
Health

WEEK
5

Healthy
Training

LESSON 17
The Rules

Task for the Day: Introduce yourself to the ground rules for a healthier living that can be implemented without a doctor's prescription.

This book doesn't intend to train you in the finer points of medicine. Turn your major injuries and illnesses over to a physician who is trained to deal with them. Corrective action for broken bones and organic breakdowns will always be a doctor's responsibility. However, basic health maintainence is in your hands. It's your job to stop problems at their source, by eliminating their causes, and to take care of little conditions early, when self-help measures will still work, before they grow serious enough to demand professional care.

We limit the discussion here to the immediate concerns of the physically active person. Some of the conditions might go unnoticed by someone less active but are important to you because they place restrictions on the quantity and quality of your activity. Some of the problems are caused by the activity and some corrected by it.

Part One of this book prescribes safe yet effective exercise programs. Part Three covers matters of dietary health. This current part deals with the causes and cures of activity-related injuries and illness.

How healthy you are depends on three sets of circumstances. Only one of them allows you much control. The first is what you're born with—heredity. You inherited certain tendencies toward health and illness from your parents, and you can't go back to reprogram your genes. A second key influence on health is where you live. Most of us endure the crowding, noise, and pollution of city and suburban living, and don't have the option to escape to a safer and more soothing environment.

What you can manage is how you live with these inherited tools and surroundings. You can make plenty of health-enhancing choices every day.

Dr. Lester Breslow of the UCLA School of Public Health has outlined the Golden Rules of healthy living. He has determined that people who regularly follow these rules can add years to their life—and, more importantly, *better* life to those years.

"The daily habits of people have a great deal more to do with what makes them sick and when they die than all the influences of medicine," says Dr. Breslow. His seven rules:

1. *Don't smoke.*
2. *Maintain normal weight.*
3. *Eat regularly and not between meals.*
4. *Eat breakfast.*
5. *Sleep seven to eight hours a night.*
6. *Drink alcohol only moderately.*
7. *Exercise consistently.*

Breslow's research indicates that a middle-aged person "who follows all seven good health habits has the same physical status as one twenty-five years younger who follows less than two of the health practices."

The order of his rules perhaps indicates that alcohol is the last vice a person will surrender, and that exercise is the last virtue one will adopt. Exercise sits at the bottom of Breslow's list, but that isn't to imply it is least important.

Dr. Nedra Belloc of the California Health Department, who worked with Breslow in the study that produced these rules, said the individuals "who reported that they engaged in active sports had the lowest mortality." Presumably, the exercisers also enjoyed the most active lives in every sense of the word.

Evidence grows that aerobic activity directly affects health in a number of beneficial ways (detailed in Lesson 19). Activity also appears to exert an indirect, catalytic effect on the other good health practices that Dr. Breslow recommends. Therefore, exercise should be given first—not last—priority among the health habits needing changing.

Thought for the Day: *How many of the Golden Rules do you follow?*

LESSON 18
The Catalyst

Task for the Day: *Start thinking of yourself as an "athlete," even if you never have competed in a sport and never will.*

Live like an athlete. Those four words sum up much of this book's advice. Living like an athlete doesn't necessarily mean training as serious competitors do, although you are asked to take scaled-down versions of their workouts. Rather, it means adopting an athletic life style.

Athletes almost automatically follow Dr. Lester Breslow's seven Golden Rules of healthy living (see Lesson 17). Training for a sport acts indirectly to promote the other good health habits.

Following a training schedule causes routines for eating and sleepng to fall into the regular patterns that Breslow recommends. People who might not have the will-power to give up cigarettes, extra helpings of dessert, or three-martini lunches—just for their health—may change their ways if athletic performance is at stake.

Studies conducted at Stanford University confirm that activity acts as a catalyst to more healthful living. Dr. Peter Wood's tests of middle-aged distance runners showed them to have physical profiles usually found only in people half their age.

Exercise has a profound effect on smoking habits. Dr. Wood reports, "Our sample of forty-five older runners contained not a single smoker, although the average number of smokers [in the United States] of similar age at the time of this study was 38 percent. However, several of them had smoked at one time when not running."

A *Runner's World* magazine survey of its readers turned up similar results. One reader in five reported smoking regularly before starting to run. Only one in *500* currently is a smoker.

In Wood's view, the non-smoking immediately gives these exercisers "an enormous health advance, since the evidence linking smoking to cancer, heart disease, and emphysema is now overwhelming."

Evidence is equally strong that obesity—gross overweight—is a drag on health. Fatness and fitness can't co-exist, and the Stanford study indicates that adult runners carry 10 percent less fat than normally inactive people their age.

"Everyone knows that exercise burns fat," says Dr. Wood. "But it takes up to fifty miles of running to burn *one pound.* Less well known is the fact that vigorous exercise regulates the appetite. This is probably the runner's secret. He or she manages to adjust caloric intake very nicely, neither wasting away nor becoming overweight."

Alcohol is "an interesting subject," according to Wood. A high percentage of the runners he studied drink it, "but I know of none of them who drink it obsessively." In other words, they seem better able to judge their limits and stay within them.

Although Dr. Wood mainly studied physiological effects of exercise, he calls the psychological effects "probably the most beneficial. Runners clearly see that powerful forces are at work, many of which act to their advantage. We know how relaxed and at peace with the world most runners are at the end of a hard run."

A group of athletic doctors would agree. The American Medical Athletic Association firmly endorses our theme of "living like an athlete."

The AMAA de-emphasizes the "don'ts" that most physicians tell patients, and which few patients follow. Instead, these doctors give one central "do." Do train for endurance.

The group's ex-president Dr. Ronald Lawrence says, "Even if it [endurance activity] didn't add a single day to a person's life, it would be worth doing—because it clearly enhances the quality of life. It changes your whole life style. You simply have more fun if smoking and drinking and other bad habits don't slow you down."

The benefits flow both ways. Changing your health habits makes athletic activity more productive, and wanting to be a better athlete makes changing habits easier.

Thought for the Day: What is more satisfying, eliminating a negative (an old habit erodes health) or adopting a positive (a new habit that will aid performance) that accomplishes the same purpose?

LESSON 19
The Effects

Task for the Day: See how far you have progressed in your exercise abilities, and why.

The human body is an amazingly pliable instrument. It adapts to almost any activity it is given, balking only to protect itself trom eventual destruction.

The responses to physical activity are standard. Everyone reacts to exercise with the same general set of adjustments. Together, they're called the "training effect."

Sudden jumps in ability by new exercisers are measurable evidence of good changes happening inside. For instance, the resting pulse rate typically drops significantly in the first few months of regular aerobic activity. This indicates more efficient heart action.

Dr. Kenneth Cooper, who has analyzed the experiences of millions of aerobic exercisers, says, "I like to think of the training effect as preventive medicine. It builds a bulwark in the body against most of the common cripplers. . . . If you've started a little late [and] one of the cripplers has already made its mark on you, the training effect can become curative medicine as well."

First, a new exerciser must clear away the effects of a sedentary life. Reduce the excess fat that has collected under the skin. Tone up the muscles. Inject more oxygen into the system. Strengthen and slow the heart. Correct degenerative problems if they haven't already progressed too far.

Even when an individual starts from what the physiologists call a "deconditioned state," the changes are often dramatic. They can be measured easily by keeping three records:

1. *Performance.* Performance includes exercise amounts and paces, as recorded in your weekly logsheets. These you should expect to improve with no increase—and often a decrease—in effort.
2. *Pulse.* The pulse should be taken while resting. A drop indicates increased efficiency of the heart as it does more work per beat.
3. *Weight.* Weigh yourself under consistent conditions (such as first thing each morning). If it was too high at the start, it almost certainly has dropped, or at least "fat weight" has been replaced by more useful and attractive "muscle weight."

These changes come with time, but they can't be rushed. They arrive only at their own pace. By trying to push it, you succeed only in driving yourself *lower* on the fitness ladder. The same activity that builds up can also tear down if taken in improper doses.

This brings us a key principle of aerobic fitness: gradual adaptation to stress. You strive to "vaccinate" yourself against the distressing aspects of this exercise. A vaccine is a small, carefully controlled dose of medicine. Taken in proper amounts, it sets up an immunity to the disease, but when taken in excess the "cure" can be worse than the ailment.

In this case, aerobic unfitness is the "disease" and activity is the vaccine. You try to build an immunity to the stresses of exercise *by exercising.* When the doses are small and their increases are carefully controlled, you grow stronger. But when the amounts of stress are excessive, you overwhelm the system's ability to adapt, thereby tearing yourself down.

Stress isn't just an emotional condition of being wound too tightly or stretched too far. And it isn't all bad. In fact, the selective application of an adaptation to physical stress lies at the heart of all training techniques. Stresses are a normal and natural part of living. They come from many directions and in various combinations (see Table 5.1). We generally absorb them into the pace of life. They become obvious and harmful only when they come in too-heavy amounts for too long a period.

Table 5.1
Stresses of Living

An active person doesn't move through a vacuum. The act of exercising is only one of many stresses at work. At least seven types of stress combine to produce a single result: the draining of adaptation reserves:

1. *Work:* Specific stress of physical activity and general stresses of the day's physical and mental labor
2. *Emotions:* Anxiety, depression, anger
3. *Social:* Isolation, overcrowding
4. *Dietary:* Improper, excessive, or inadequate food; drug abuse
5. *Rest:* Incomplete recovery from hard work; sleep deprivation
6. *Health:* Injury, illness, infection
7. *Environment:* Heat, cold, air pollution

Overstressing causes many illnesses and injuries. They are often self-inflicted, and therefore can be self-corrected.

The signs and symptoms of excessive stress are easy to spot (Week 6 covers them in detail). Detecting and correcting the causes early help to minimize damage. But if stress loads remain too high, they eventually lead to serious complications.

Dr. Hans Selye, a Canadian medical researcher, made the stress phenomenon his life's work. He observed that every disease is a symptom of stress that a person can't handle, and that many of the physical breakdowns of exercisers come from this same source. "When we finished our laborious analysis of its nature," says Dr. Selye, "stress turned out to be something quite simple to understand. It is essentially the wear and tear in the body caused by life at any one time."

Selye notes that a person exposed to this wear and tear erects defenses to counteract it. The body has a reservoir of "adaptive energy" for handling everyday battering, plus a reserve supply for emergencies.

But if the doses of stress are too heavy and prolonged, the individual can no longer adapt or even cope. The reserves are drained, and he or she goes into what Selye calls the "exhaustion phase of the General Adaptation Syndrome" (GAS). Symptoms then appear. Among the most common are lingering fatigue, colds and fever, and muscle or tendon pain. (These are discussed in Week 6.)

According to Selye, "When superficial adaptation energy is exhausted through exertion, it can slowly be restored from a deeper store during rest." The doctor warns that each time a person ignores stress symptoms and digs deeper into emergency energy supplies, he or she risks major damage.

So how does all this theory translate into practical terms for a physically active person? Avoid stress? Not at all. If you're trying to improve as an exerciser, you must seek it out and travel a thin line between enough and too much.

Think of yourself as a violin string. Like the string, you have a great performance capacity. But that potential is wasted when you lie limp and unused. Only when you're stretched are you filling your intended role. But that stretching can go too far. When pressures pull too hard in opposite directions, *snap!* The trick is to find a point of stretch or stress, a level of activity, that makes music while holding resiliency in reserve. When emergencies come up—either real, as unavoidable life crises, or artificial, in the form of hard training—you then should be able to meet them by stretching more instead of snapping.

Dr. Hans Selye concludes, "The goal is certainly not to avoid stress. Stress is a part of life. It is a natural by-product of all-out activity.

"There is no more justification for avoiding stress than for shunning food, exercise, or love. But in order to express yourself fully, you must find your optimum stress level."

Thought for the Day: How well are you bearing up your total stress load?

LESSON 20
The Calories

Task for the Day: Find a new way to count calories—not as amount eaten but expended.

Dr. Ralph Paffenbarger's specialty is epidemiology. The Stanford University professor studies large groups of people for long periods of time.

An early project of his followed longshoremen for more than twenty years. Those who labored hardest were shown to run only half the heart attack risk of those who had easier jobs.

Another Paffenbarger study dealt with a much different group: Harvard University graduates from the first half of this century. In the 1960s, he mailed questionnaires to 36,000 alumni. They were asked their exercise habits and disease patterns. Nearly 17,000 of them responded. In the early 1970s, Dr. Paffenbarger sent follow-up questionnaires to these men. About 600 of them had suffered heart attacks in the meantime.

The victims, he learned, were more likely to be the non-exercisers. This wasn't surprising; the connection had been suspected for some time. What surprised the medical community was how clearly this study pointed out the benefits of vigorous exercise. *

---

*Running and walking each consume about 100 calories per mile. But Paffenbarger doesn't say you must train twenty or more miles each week. Other, incidental daily exercise counts toward this total. See a more detailed listing of caloric costs of various exercises in Week 10.

Paffenbarger used the number of calories burned as his measuring stick. He identified 2,000 a week as the dividing line between light and heavy exercise.

Harvard alumni who exercised less than this amount had 64 percent more heart attacks than those who worked harder at staying in shape. Putting it another way, Dr. Paffenbarger said that if all the men had exercised at or above the 2,000-calorie weekly level, 166 more of them would have avoided heart attacks.

He anticipated two challenges to this research: that other factors in a person's life may have been responsible for this protection, and that those men most attracted to hard exercise were least likely to develop heart disease in the first place.

To the first challenge, Paffenbarger responded that the protection given by strenuous physical activity was "largely independent" of other risk factors such as smoking, high blood pressure, and family history of heart disease.

He also rejected the claim that exercisers were safer at the beginning. Former varsity athletes were as susceptible to heart disease as non-athletes after they quit training. Yet those who took up vigorous sports for the first time as adults enjoyed full protection.

Dr. Paffenbarger's case for exercise has gained strength over the years. He found after reviewing new data in the mid-1980s that Harvard alumni who regularly exercised at or above the 2,000-calorie-a-week total "had a 30 percent lower death rate than those who hardly exercised." This study, he said, "adds new evidence to support the view that physical exercise preserves life and its desirable qualities."

The first signs of physical degeneration were found in men who exercised away fewer than 500 calories a week. Exercisers at the 3,500-plus level declined the slowest. People who trained at this level were less than half as likely to die prematurely than those who stayed inactive. Going beyond 3,500 calories, however, produced diminishing returns. Apparently, a point comes in exercising for life when the cost of straining begins to outweigh the benefits of training.

To reach his 2,000-calorie minimum, Dr. Paffenbarger suggested taking several hours a week of vigorous activity. Running, walking, swimming, and bicycling lead his list of exercises. He said with scientific certainty, "We can expect that for every hour exercisers are active, they will get to live that hour over—and maybe two more on top of that—later in life."

Thought for the Day: How many calories do you spend each week as life insurance?

Now look at Table 5.2 to log in your training time for the week.

Table 5.2
Week 5 Training Chart

Record your physical training for the week, including only formal sessions, not incidental daily exercise. List the actual date, aerobic activity, duration in minutes, and any supplemental "muscle" exercises. A suggested weekly program would include four aerobic training days, lasting at least 30 minutes, with not more than two training days in a row or more than two straight rest days.

Day (Date)	Aerobic Exercise	Duration	Other Exercise
Sunday			
Monday			
Tuesday			
Wednesday			
Thursday			
Friday			
Saturday			

Total aerobic training time for the week: _____

Number of aerobic sessions: _____

Average time per session: _____

WEEK
6

Medical Care

LESSON 21
The Causes

Task for the Day: Identify the most common source of an aerobic exerciser's ailments.

This is not a pleasant subject, but it's one that every exerciser must face occasionally: What happens when you can't train as often, as fast, or as long as you'd like due to injury or illness?

Trouble can ambush you from many directions. These include accidents (the result of bad luck, some of which you may create), the environment (ill effects of heat and cold, among others) and faulty equipment (notably for the on-foot exerciser, improper shoes).

We'll get to all of these matters in Week 7. For now, the subject is a category that gives aerobic exercisers more problems than all the other causes combined: training errors. You generally inflict these conditions on yourself.

Unfortunately, exercise is not perfectly safe. It is work, and it can easily cross the line into *overwork*. People seeking the thrill of victory (if only over their own unfitness) often experience the agony of defeat—in the form of inactivity from stress-induced breakdowns.

The injury rates from seemingly nonviolent aerobic activities can be high. In any year, for example, one runner in every two is hurt badly enough to require a layoff, medical treatment, or both. Most of these injuries are self-inflicted. They result neither from a competitor's blows (as might happen in football), nor from a random accident, (such as hitting a rock while skiing), nor from bad equipment (wrong shoes). The stress of the activity itself takes the blame in a high percentage of cases.

Most of these injuries also are so minor that a non-exerciser wouldn't even notice them. They heal quickly and completely with treatment as simple as rest or the temporary substitution of a less stressful activity. Certain viruses such as the common cold and the flu afflict exercisers in similar ways. You're constantly exposed to these illnesses, yet they rarely surface unless stress has broken down the body's natural defenses.

The great majority of medical conditions that slow or stop aerobic activity grow out of what the sports doctors call "overuse": too much wear and tear on a body not conditioned to handle so much stress. In this fact lies hope. Because you cause most of your own ailments, you also have the power to prevent them. The damage doesn't often strike randomly. Athletic ailments aren't punishment from the wrathful gods, but are predictable results of too much work and too little attention to obvious warnings. You hold the power to prevent this kind of trouble.

Dr. Hans Selye was never a serious athlete. Yet the Canadian medical researcher provided a basis for modern training with his General Adaptation Syndrome (GAS) theories (detailed in Week 5). To review, Selye argues that a person exposed to stress (physical exercise is one stress among many) erects defenses to counteract it. If you apply the stress in small, regular doses, the body adapts to it by growing stronger. But if the doses are too heavy, the body can't cope. It goes into the "exhaustion" phase, becoming susceptible to physical breakdowns.

The trick in physical training, then, is to exercise enough to build but not so much that you tear down. The same activity can be helpful or hurtful, depending on how you apply it.

How do you determine the right amount? Adaptive success and failure are fairly easy to detect. Improved performance accompanied by pain-free activity indicate that you're adapting nicely to this stress. On the other hand, your body sends out danger signals as you approach the exhausted state. Develop a sensitive "eye" to these signals. By reading and interpreting them, you go a long way toward stopping trouble at its source.

When the stress load grows too heavy, for whatever reason, certain mild symptoms appear. Those listed in Table 6.1 warn that more serious trouble might develop if you don't take immediate preventive action.

Table 6.1
Warning Signs

Prevention of injuries and illnesses usually involves reducing or eliminating stresses (listed in Table 5.1). One of the most flexible is your training load. Adjust it whenever any of the following warning signs appear:

1. Resting pulse rate significantly higher than normal when taken first thing in the morning
2. Sudden, dramatic loss of weight
3. Difficulty falling asleep and staying asleep
4. Sores in and around the mouth, and other skin eruptions in non-adolescents
5. Any symptom of a cold or the flu: sniffles, sore throat, or fever
6. Swollen, tender glands in the neck, groin, or underarms
7. Labored breathing during the mild exertion of a physical training session
8. Dizziness or nausea before, during, or after training
9. Clumsiness—for instance, tripping or kicking yourself during a run over rather smooth ground
10. Any muscle, tendon, or joint pain or stiffness that remains after the first few minutes of exercise

---

Thought for the Day: Would you rather pay attention to these symptoms now, or pay later for ignoring them?

LESSON 22
The Injuries

Task for the Day: Learn how exercisers get hurt, how badly, and how long they stay that way.

An aerobic exerciser's injury doesn't usually strike with sudden and devastating consequences, like a compound fracture of the leg. These problems are more in the nature of slow, steady erosion that wears down the body.

The physical pain of most exercise-induced injuries doesn't even amount to much—hurting less than an average headache or toothache, if at all, when you're at rest. However, a sore spot the size of a dime can be debilitating when you put full weight on it.

Annual surveys by *Runner's World* magazine tell the type and frequency of these problems. More than half of the runners surveyed were injured badly enough within the past year to curtail training, visit a doctor, or both. (Note that these people often were serious athletes, and their casualty rates probably far exceed those of more conservative exercisers.)

This survey also included the following findings:

- The weakest link in runners is the knee. About one in five of them has suffered a knee injury.
- Nearly as many break down at the Achilles tendon, the thin band of tissue connecting the heel bone with the calf muscles.
- Ten percent suffer "shin splints," an imprecise term covering ailments at the front of the lower leg. These range from tendinitis to stress fractures.
- Forefoot strains and stress fractures, heel pain, and damage to the arch each account for about 7 percent of injuries.

Muscle tears in the legs and problems higher up, with the hips and lower back, are more rare in runners. The risks of running have led some former specialists to vary their activities. This "cross-training," or blending various aerobic activities, has become a popular practice during the 1980s. Many exercisers choose the triathlon mixture of running, bicycling, and swimming.

Cross-training has much to recommend it. But its role in injury prevention may be overrated. That appears to be true, anyway, when this mix leads to serious triathlon training and competition. In 1986 researchers at Mount Sinai Medical Center in New York City compared the injury rates of triathletes against those of specialists in the component sports: swimmers, cyclists, and runners. In a one-year period, swimming produced a 33-percent casualty rate; bicycling, 51 percent, and running, 61. The figure for triathloning: *90 percent.*

Commenting on this report, Dr. George Sheehan speculates that so many triathletes get hurt because they pile the stresses from all three activities on top of each other. "Cross-training works only if total training time is not increased," says Dr. Sheehan. "Otherwise the additional training time will result in more overall injuries."

The Mount Sinai study also revealed that triathletes were most often hurt while they ran, causing Sheehan to note that "running is the chief hazard to the triathlete, just as it is to the runner."

In other words, less emphasis on the run might have kept triathletes healthier. Turning over some of the training time to biking and swimming might do the same for runners.

This research found that the running group's injuries healed slowest. Their average time to complete recovery was forty days, compared to twenty-seven days for triathletes, and less than two weeks for swimmers and cyclists.

These injured runners couldn't run at all on twenty-five of those rehabilitation days. That was when they might have substituted a less painful activity. Cross-training serves its best purpose by reducing downtime.

Thought for the Day: What would you do if an injury took away your favorite activity?

LESSON 23
The Recovery

Task for the Day: Plan an alternative route to aerobic fitness in case touble develops.

An injury has knocked you off your feet. What to do now? Whatever the specific problem is, the road back to health follows a similar path. It allows you to heal while staying somewhat active.

This recovery course starts with a few "don'ts":

- *Don't make a bad problem worse* by trying to train through pain. Attempt nothing that causes you to limp or "favor" the injured area.
- *Don't worry about losing fitness.* If you developed it over months and years, it won't disappear in days or weeks.
- *Don't take an all-or-nothing approach.* Instead of giving up your training routine completely if you can't practice it all, mimic it with alternate or modified activity.

Choose an exercise that doesn't aggravate the problem. Then train at the normal time of day and for the normal period of time. For instance, if you normally would run and can't do so without limping, mix walking and running. If all running is impossible, just walk. If walking hurts too much, bike or swim. As recovery allows, work up the exercise ladder by the following steps:

1. *Biking or swimming.* These activities take nearly all the pressure off most foot and leg injuries, while still giving steady training. They allow you to keep the demons of self-doubt at bay.
2. *Walking.* Start it as soon as you can move without "favoring" the injured limb. Continue as long as pain doesn't become intense. (These limitations apply at all stages.)
3. *Walking mixed with running.* As the walks become too easy, add brief periods of easy running—as little as one minute in five at first, then gradually building up the amount of running.
4. *Running mixed with walking.* Keep inserting brief walking breaks—say, one minute in five—while steady pressure can't yet be tolerated.

5. *Running again.* Approach it cautiously for a while—a little slower than normal until typical daily runs can be handled comfortably.

(A similar plan, minus stage one, can ease you back into training after a prolonged illness—or after a voluntary layoff during which your fitness has suffered.)

Dr. David Brody, a sports-medicine specialist from Washington, D.C., has a ready answer for runners who ask, ''What can I do to keep from losing all my fitness when I'm injured and can't run?''

Dr. Brody tells them to run exactly as they had before—but to do it in deep water, wearing a water-ski vest to protect the injury. This isn't vague, untested advice.

Brody studied eight runners for the training benefits of water-running. They volunteered to stop training on land for eight weeks, and to substitute ''runs'' of equal time and intensity in the deep end of a pool. They finished the test by running the Marine Corps Marathon in Washington. All of the subjects improved their previous best times for this distance—after two months off the roads.

Dr. Brody warns, however, that these athletes were marathon-trained before the study began. Someone with little or no such background probably couldn't expect to *get* in shape with this substitute activity. But it is an excellent way to *stay* fit when you must be off your feet.

Thought for the Day: What would be your second and third choices of exercise if you couldn't practice the main one?

LESSON 24
The Illnesses

Task for the Day: Find ways to treat the common cold and to play it cool with a fever.

A common cold is nature's way of telling you to relax. You don't so much catch it as it *catches you* when your defenses are down. Overstressing yourself leaves you vulnerable to this ever-present virus that you normally might fight off.

Exercise sometimes makes some people ill—literally. But it can also act as preventive medicine or an aid to treatment. It all depends on how you use it or abuse it.

The good news first: Evidence gleaned from several scientific studies indicates that vigorous aerobic exercisers such as runners suffer fewer colds, as a group, than non-exercisers. This apparently has to do with normally increased body heat, which may destroy some of the ''bugs.'' However, continued hard work in the face of early symptoms can turn a mild cold into a dreadful one, and may lead to side effects such as bronchitis. Coming down with a cold means you already have worked too hard. Don't compound the problem.

Dr. George Sheehan, a sports-medicine columnist for several magazines, spends a large part of each month counseling ailing exercisers. Here is a summary of his advice for handling this most common of illnesses:

"I treat it with respect. It is my feeling that it represents a breakdown in the defense system. The cold is an early warning of exhaustion." Dr. Sheehan advises heeding your body's warnings, and cutting back or even cutting out training for the first one to three days of the cold. "Then resume at a slow pace for relatively short distances." He recommends not waiting for all symptoms to subside. Moderate exercise in the waning stages of the illness, says Sheehan, helps clear away the lingering congestion.

Dr. Terry Kavanagh, a Canadian who pioneered the use of aerobic exercise for heart patients (including those receiving transplants), is more lenient than Sheehan. Dr. Kavanagh says, "If it's a common cold without a fever, mild exercise may shorten the duration of the cold." The key words here are *moderate, mild,* and *fever.* Exhaustion led, at least in part, to contracting this illness. Therefore, avoiding further exhausting efforts is your best medicine.

"Don't run with a fever," warns Dr. George Sheehan of this condition most commonly associated with the flu. "Rest until it passes. After that, as a rule of thumb, take two days easy for each day of fever. A week of fever and symptoms, therefore, would need an additional two weeks' recovery period. Exhausting workouts should be avoided at this time, or recurrence of the illness is a distinct possibility."

This advice can't be emphasized too strongly. Ignoring it can lead to severe complications, including heart problems.

Dr. David Bewick, a cardiologist from Canada, noticed that the flu temporarily affected the heart in nearly all of the patients he studied. "Our findings suggest that cardiac involvement in the various viral syndromes may be tissue-specific," said Dr. Bewick in a report to the American Heart Association, "with influenza affecting mainly the myocardium." (This is heart tissue.) Bewick added, "Our people were young and at the very mild end of the spectrum, and when the viral infection subsided, their hearts got back to normal." He warned against trying to "run off" the illness.

An example of where that might lead comes from a high-level source. Steve Ovett, a former world record-holder in track, recalls what happened to him before, during and long after the 1984 Olympic Games. "I had the flu," says the British runner. "But with the Games coming up, I trained through my illness and thought I was over it. In Los Angeles, I knew something was wrong. The harder I pushed, the worse the pains in my chest got. I had all the classic symptoms of a heart attack, and finally my body just quit." He dropped out of the 1,500-meter final.

Complications slowed his recovery. "It wasn't until well after the Games," Ovett recalls, "that I learned I had pericarditis, a viral infection of the sac covering the heart. It took me five months to recover fully."

Dr. Terry Kavanagh gives this advice: "If you have a fever, usually associated with the flu, stop all exercise. The body can't cope with the double stress. I tell people to wait until they are fully recovered from the flu, and then add five days before they begin [exercising] again."

Even if the training does no harm, nothing is gained from it. The body is crying for time off from work of all kinds.

Thought for the Day: What would you do, and not do, if you had a cold or the flu?

Now turn to Table 6.2 to log in your training time for the week.

Table 6.2
Week 6 Training Chart

Record your physical training for the week, including only formal sessions, not incidental daily exercise. List the actual date, aerobic activity, duration in minutes, and any supplemental "muscle" exercises. A suggested weekly program would include four aerobic training days, lasting at least 30 minutes, with not more than two training days in a row or more than two straight rest days.

Day (Date)	Aerobic Exercise	Duration	Other Exercise
Sunday			
Monday			
Tuesday			
Wednesday			
Thursday			
Friday			
Saturday			

Total aerobic training time for the week: _____

Number of aerobic sessions: _____

Average time per session: _____

WEEK
7

Safe
Travels

LESSON 25
The Threats

Task for the Day: Be aware of the risks facing outdoor exercisers.

Dr. George Sheehan once remarked with tongue only partly in cheek that runners have three natural enemies: "dogs, drivers, and doctors." He explained that each group seems bent on taking the activity. Dogs attack, drivers rule the roads, and some doctors say, "It hurts to run? Then don't run."

Fortunately, the medical profession has come to realize that what aerobic exercisers want most is to keep exercising. Led by pioneers such as Sheehan, doctors now provide solid information on avoiding and treating injuries, rather than dispensing simplistic "stop-doing-it" advice.

This one-time adversary is now converted to friend. Yapping dogs are more a nuisance than a threat. Our concern here is with the true enemies— those with the power to exert deadly force either accidentally (in traffic) or intentionally (at the hands of an attacker).

ACCIDENTS

Streets and roads are convenient places to run/walk, and you probably do much of your training there. They offer smooth, all-weather surfaces. In town, the streets are lighted for early morning and late evening exercise. You hit the roads for convenience, and in doing so court their dangers.

Training in traffic is by far the greatest exercise risk you face. Look at the odds: You take perhaps 150 pounds of soft flesh to the road and travel less than 8 miles an hour. The automobile weighs more than ten times that much, may travel ten times as fast, and is made of hard metal. When pedestrian meets car, the loser is obvious.

The Insurance Institute for Highway Safety (1982) analyzed sixty runner/auto accidents occurring during a one-year period. Half of the runners died of their injuries. When police assessed the blame for the collisions, nearly half were equally the fault of the driver and the runner. Nineteen cases were charged to runner error and sixteen to the driver.

Questions of blame are academic, and the idea that the pedestrian has the right-of-way is strictly a legal principle. Too many of the victims wind up dead right. If you choose to use the roads as your training ground, please observe these common sense precautions listed in Table 7.1.

Table 7.1
Road Safety

1. When training on the streets or road, always yield the right of way. The roads belong to the vehicles because of their size. Don't challange them for space, because you'll lose any such argument.
2. Run/walk defensively and with a hint of paranoia. Assume that all drivers are out to get you, and don't give them that chance.
3. Stay awake. Fight the tendency to daydream away the miles. Keep your head up and eyes on the road.
4. Be seen, particularly when training in the dark. Wear brightly colored clothing in the daytime and reflective items at night.
5. See what's coming. Wear a visor or billed cap in darkness to shade your eyes from headlights that could blind you. (Drivers rarely dim their lights for oncoming pedestrians.)
6. Hear what's coming. Leave your cassette tape player or earphone radio at home if the music might drown out warnings of danger.
7. Be most careful at sunrise and sunset. Several factors make these the most dangerous hours: rush hour traffic, sleepy or exhausted commuters, and the glare of the low sun in the driver's or your eyes.
8. Use sidewalks whenever possible. When using the roadway, stay on the right, facing traffic—except when that side offers little room and the left appears safer.
9. Don't ignore bicycles and motorcycles. They travel almost as fast as cars, are less visible, and can inflict great damage both to you and the rider.
10. Don't provoke drivers by invading their lane, darting across in front of them, or pounding their cars in cases of close calls. A car can be a deadly weapon in the hands of an angry driver.

ATTACKS

Humans armed with hostility sometimes pose risks to you. Women suffer most in this regard, both in number of victims and through restrictions placed on their free movement. Most attackers choose women as targets for their verbal and even physical abuse. These incidents are distressingly common, and the consequences can be most serious.

In 1981 RunHers, a women's running club in Washington, DC, reported shocking data on threats and attacks directed at its members. Of ninety-nine women questioned, forty-one reported one or more incidents. Most of these were verbal harassment, but more than one-quarter of the cases involved being chased or grabbed.

Laura MacKenzie, who compiled the report, noted, "No area is completely safe. Vigilance is always prudent. However, some types of areas are considerably safer than others."

Neighborhoods appear safest. RunHers members trained 38 percent of the time in residential areas, but only 16 percent of incidents occurred there. The risk increases on bike paths. These were the scene of 25 percent of the problems, while these women ran there 21 percent of the time.

Parks are most dangerous. Only 6 percent of training was done in secluded parklands, but this setting accounted for *27 percent* of the threats and attacks.

This report points out the greatest inequity in public exercising: Men can train alone almost anywhere at anytime, while the options available to a lone woman are much more limited. Women fight back several ways. They train in pairs and groups for safety in numbers, they restrict their activities to daylight hours, or they carry weapons such as chemical sprays. All of these systems work, but none is entirely satisfactory if the woman wants both solitary effort and peace of mind.

Perhaps the best solution is to exercise with a big dog. "I haven't had a single comment from a guy since I began running with my Doberman pinscher," says one woman who had been bothered frequently before. "The main thing dogs have going for them as partners that people don't is the dog will run at your time and your convenience, your pace and your distance, without expecting you to carry on a witty conversation."

Thought for the Day: *How do you put a safe distance between yourself and danger?*

LESSON 26
The Earth

Task for the Day: *Check the benefits and risks of various running/walking surfaces and terrains.*

SURFACE

A running magazine's survey unmasked a myth—one that says pounding along on hard surfaces is most likely to produce injuries, while soft surfaces such as grass and dirt are kindest to the feet and legs. A *Runner's World* study (1979) involving thousands of runners indicated that those who trained on grass and dirt got hurt just as often as those who ran entirely on asphalt and concrete. The conclusion was that errors in training routine are more likely than the running surface to cause problems.

Improvements in shoes (see Lesson 27) have neutralized much of the pounding, and most runners/walkers now use the roads for reasons noted in Lesson 25: they generally are lighted for exercising at any hour, they are usable in all weather conditions, and they offer sure, smooth footing.

While practicalities dictate that much of your training will be on hard surfaces, don't deprive yourself completely of the softer ones. The study quoted above ignores one key fact: Minor aches (as opposed to true injuries) from constant pounding are clearly greater on hard road surfaces, and the soft ones are more pleasing aesthetically.

TERRAIN

Hills make for harder work, whether the surface is soft or unyielding.

Hills are a stress that a beginning exerciser doesn't need. They add extra stresses that he or she isn't yet prepared to handle. Hills send pulse and breathing rates to their peaks, well past ideal aerobic training levels. Hills, both up and down, also put extra strain on legs that still aren't fully conditioned.

As a general rule, stay off steep hills completely until you can run a half-hour or walk a full hour on the flat. After graduating to hills, give them the respect they deserve. They shrink for no one, so you have to do the adapting.

Adjust to running and walking in the hills as you would while riding a ten-speed bicycle on hilly terrain. You wouldn't ride up and down in the same gear used on the flat. You'd shift, pump, coast, and brake in tune with the slope—all the while maintaining a constant pedaling rate.

Shift to lower "gears" while running/walking uphill. Cut the stride length. Lean into the hill a bit. Try to keep the *effort* fairly constant, which means reducing the pace.

While going downhill, shift into a higher "gear." Lean forward slighly to take advantage of gravity. Don't be too proud to do some braking to keep from racing out of control.

Thought for the Day: *Are you ready to head for the hills and equipped for the hard ground?*

LESSON 27
The Shoes

Task for the Day: *Study the on-foot exerciser's most important item of equipment.*

Splurge on good shoes—running or walking shoes and not those designed for other activities. These shoes are rather expensive and are growing more so. But they are a most important investment, not a luxury. Your health and performance rest on your feet, so protect them well. Plan on spending about $40 to $50 for a good pair of shoes. This will be your only major, recurring equipment expense.

What to look for in shoes? First, consider your needs. You probably are training modest amounts at modest paces, not trying to race a mile or finish a marathon.

If you have recently started to exercise, you may be somewhat heavier than you'd prefer. Your feet and legs may not be conditioned to tolerate the pounding inflicted by hard surfaces. Therefore, look for well-cushioned, well-supported shoes (but not excessively so on either count) with the following features:

- A soft, nonirritating upper material. Nylon or suede is softer than standard leather.
- Adequate toe room, both in terms of length and height. This is a function of size and the cut of the shoe.
- Firm sole material on the outside for durability and a softer midsole for comfort.
- Heel lift, a wedge that raises the heel about a quarter to a half-inch higher than the sole.
- Heel support in the form of rigid material around the back for stability.
- Forefoot flexibility so the foot can bend easily.

Many well-established manufacturers stand ready to fill these needs. In alphabetical order, the best-selling brands are Adidas, Asics (formerly Tiger), Avia, Brooks, Converse, Etonic, New Balance, Nike, Puma, Reebok, and Saucony. Choose shoes from these companies, and you can't go far wrong. Examine the properties of other brands more closely.

Prices vary enormously. You can pick up minor brands in discount stores for less than $20, and you can buy high-tech models for $100 or more. Avoid both extremes. You can protect yourself adequately with name-brand shoes costing $30 to $60.

Another consideration is your foot type. Doctors specializing in foot health categorize feet as "floppy" and "rigid." The first tends to be flat, while the second shows extremely high arches. The floppy foot needs greater stability from shoes (the tradeoffs are reduced cushioning and flexibility). The rigid foot requires more cushioning, more flexibility. Figure 7.1 illustrates the types of shoes that best meet these needs.

The first step in avoiding equipment-related injury is making the right shoe choice. The second step is not letting these shoes wear out too much. All shoes break down from hard use, losing cushioning and support as well as sole material. The critical factor is excessive wear at the heels, which can tip you out of balance and lead to injuries. When a quarter- to a half-inch of heel is gone, consider repairing or replacing the shoes. Your feet and legs will thank you.

Thought for the Day: *How good were your shoes when new, and what is their condition now?*

LESSON 28
The Air

Task for the Day: *Learn to live with hot and cold weather.*

As an outdoor exerciser, you don't need a weatherman to know which way the wind blows. You live with the elements, and probably taste the extremes of heat and cold. An important fact to recognize when dealing with these elements is the difference between standing in the heat or cold, and exercising under the same conditions. Heat often intensifies during exercise, while cold tends to lose some if its sting. These effects are most pronounced in running and occur to a lesser extent during other activities.

HEAT

Exercising on a hot day increases the body's heat production, so a nice afternoon for suntanning beside the pool may be a difficult one for training. For

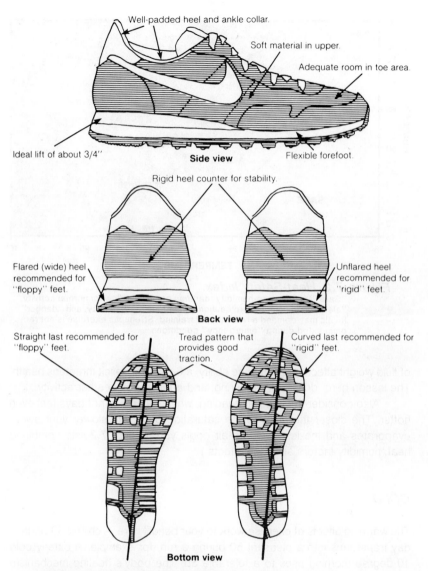

Figure 7.1 Anatomy of a Shoe

instance, a 20-degree rule applies to running. The perceived temperature automatically rises by that much in the course of a run. So a nice, sunny, 70-degree afternoon soon feels like a steamy 90°.

The body acts on what it feels, not what the thermometer reads. As internal heat goes up, you compensate by sweating and can only sweat so much before dehydration sets in. In Week 8, you'll learn that a 3-percent loss

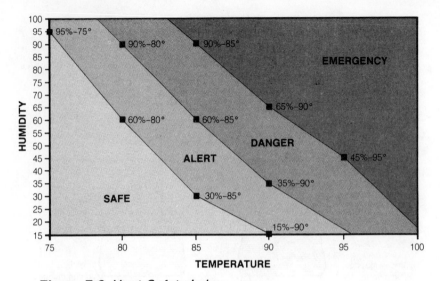

Figure 7.2 *Heat-Safety Index.*
"Safe" temperature-humidity readings generally allow for normal activity, "alert" conditions require caution during long, hard activity, and "danger" levels may demand a reduction of training. Strenuous exercise is not recommended during "emergency" conditions.

of fluid weight affects performance ability: a 6-percent deficit threatens health. The lesson here: drink before, during, and after all hot-weather activity.

Also consider the humidity reading, which can make hot days feel even hotter. The closer the air is to the saturation point, the slower your sweat evaporates and the less well the air cools you. (Figure 7.2 lists combined heat/humidity factors and their effects.)

COLD

The warming effects of exercise work to your benefit here. A chilling 30-degree day transforms into a pleasant 50 during a run, for example. A bitterly cold 10-degree morning rises to a tolerable 30. The body's heating mechanism that makes you miserable on hot days can make running more comfortable on cold ones. At all but the extremes of low temperature and high wind, you warm up adequately if you're well dressed.

Humidity makes summer weather unbearable. In winter, it's the wind. Temperatures feel colder than the thermometer shows on windy days. Each mile per hour of wind drops the apparent temperature by about 1 degree. Wind-chills below minus 20 degrees carry "increased danger" of frostbite, and those below minus 70 pose "great danger" (see Figure 7.3).

Temperature (Fahrenheit)

Equivalent Chill Temperature

Wind speed (miles per hour)	Calm	40	35	30	25	20	15	10	5	0	−5	−10	−15	−20	−25	−30	−35	−40	−45	−50	−55	−60
Calm		40	35	30	25	20	15	10	5	0	−5	−10	−15	−20	−25	−30	−35	−40	−45	−50	−55	−60
5		35	30	25	20	15	10	5	0	−5	−10	−15	−20	−25	−30	−35	−40	−45	−50	−55	−65	−70
10		30	20	15	10	5	0	−10	−15	−20	−25	−35	−40	−45	−50	−60	−65	−70	−75	−80	−90	−95
15		25	15	10	0	−5	−10	−20	−25	−30	−40	−45	−50	−60	−65	−70	−80	−85	−90	−100	−105	−110
20		20	10	5	0	−10	−15	−25	−30	−35	−45	−50	−60	−65	−75	−80	−85	−95	−100	−110	−115	−120
25		15	10	0	−5	−15	−20	−30	−35	−45	−50	−60	−65	−75	−80	−90	−95	−105	−110	−120	−125	−135
30		10	5	0	−10	−20	−25	−30	−40	−50	−55	−65	−70	−80	−85	−95	−100	−110	−115	−120	−130	−140
35		10	5	−5	−10	−20	−30	−35	−40	−50	−60	−65	−75	−80	−90	−100	−105	−115	−120	−130	−135	−145
40*		10	0	−5	−15	−20	−30	−35	−45	−55	−60	−70	−75	−85	−95	−100	−110	−115	−125	−130	−140	−150

— Little Danger

Increasing Danger
(Flesh may freeze
within one minute)

Great Danger
(Flesh may freeze
within 30 seconds)

*Winds above 40 m.p.h. have little additional effect.

Figure 7.3 Wind-Chill Readings

On typical winter days, there is little risk of frostbite if you keep moving and have your hands and ears covered. There is even less danger of "freezing the lungs" from breathing icy air. If the air had that much feared effect, would any skiers survive the slopes or skaters the outdoor rinks?

CLOTHING

Dress for function, not fashion—for comfort and the conditions not for show. One of the beauties of the simplest aerobic activities are their low cost. Don't neutralize it by outfitting yourself as if you were headed for a style show.

The central guideline on clothing has to do with the weather: *Don't over-dress.* The tendency among people inexperienced with exercise at the extremes of weather is to dress for comfort while standing still. They heat up inside while training, and wish they'd left half of their clothes at home. Leave that half there before going out, or dress in layers (a jacket over a sweater over a T-shirt on a cold day) that can be easily stripped off en route.

If you're walking or running, dress for temperatures up to 20 degrees warmer than they seem at the start. Generally speaking, a hot day for running is one when the temperature exceeds 70, warm is in the 50 to 60 range, cool is just above freezing through the high 40s, and cold is below freezing. (These figures are, of course, skewed by the effects of high humidity in hot weather and wind-chill factors on cold days. See Figures 7.2 and 7.3.)

Start dressing each day from a foundation of underwear, socks, shoes, and shorts. Add layers from a basic wardrobe including the following items: a sleeveless tank top (on hot days); long pants and long-sleeved shirt (for cold weather); jacket, gloves, and stocking cap (for cold conditions).

Rain needn't stop you. Just add a baseball-style cap or visor to keep the water off your face, wear rain-repelling clothing if the day is cool, and splash away. Think of it this way: You're already wet from sweat, so the rain can't make you much wetter. (Figure 7.4 illustrates clothing needs for various conditions.)

Thought for the Day: *What effect does the day's weather report have on your plans to exercise?*

Now turn to Table 7.2 to log in your training time for the week.

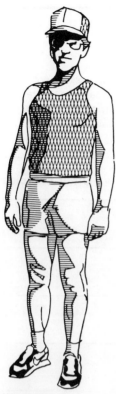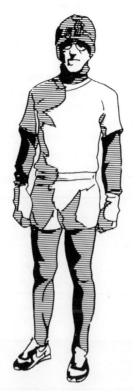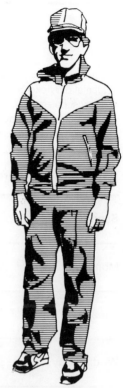

Hot weather
Dress in minimal light-colored clothing (such as mesh baseball style cap, mesh top) that both protects from the sun and "breathes."

Cold weather
Dress in several layers of clothing, for instance, tights and turtleneck shirt under shorts and T-shirt; and gloves and stocking cap to protect head and hands.

Wet, cool weather
Dress in light, rain-repellent clothing. Wear baseball style cap to keep rain out of face. Gloves are optional.

Figure 7.4 Clothes for All Seasons

Table 7.2
Week 7 Training Chart

Record your physical training for the week, including only formal sessions, not incidental daily exercise. List the actual date, aerobic activity, duration in minutes, and any supplemental "muscle" exercises. A suggested weekly program would include four aerobic training days, lasting at least 30 minutes, with not more than two training days in a row or more than two straight rest days.

Day (Date)	Aerobic Exercise	Duration	Other Exercise
Sunday			
Monday			
Tuesday			
Wednesday			
Thursday			
Friday			
Saturday			

Total aerobic training time for the week: _____

Number of aerobic sessions: _____

Average time per session: _____

PART
Three

Your
Diet

WEEK
8

Dietary
Training

Task for the Day: Introduce yourself to the requirements of everyone who eats and drinks.

The best way to preview sound athletic nutrition is first to talk about sound *human* nutrition. The endurance athlete's or aerobic exerciser's basic needs aren't very different from those of any other healthy person. We're all bound by the same broad dietary rules.

Today, you learn some of those general laws. They provide a necessary framework for understanding the specifics of the active person's diet (contained in this chapter and in Weeks 9 and 10). This isn't meant to be a complete course in nutrition, only an introduction put in simplest terms. Some factors are skipped over lightly or are ignored completely—either because they're too obvious to mention or have little direct bearing on your activity.

Everything we take in by mouth and send on the long, complex trip through the digestive system serves one or more of the following purposes: energy production (providing fuel for work), growth (building and repairing tissues), and control (regulating body processes).

Six classes of nutrients do these jobs:

1. *Carbohydrates*. These are the high-energy foods, primarily sugars and starches. Their energy characteristics give them utmost importance in the athletic context. In relatively short, fast bursts of effort, carbohydrate products are the main fuel source because they can be used quickly and efficiently.

2. *Fats.* Because of the connection with obesity and heart disease, fats have gotten a bad name. In fact, animal fats and vegetable oils are another essential energy source. During heavy exercise, however, fats go to work slower than carbohydrates.

3. *Proteins.* These are the body-builders, helping bones and tissues grow and repair themselves, and the body needs regular amounts of protein to keep operating well. Its most obvious forms are meat, fish, and fowl. However, protein needs can be met entirely without eating animal flesh. Eggs, dairy products, nuts, beans, peas, and grains also supply this nutrient.

4. *Minerals.* To the aerobic exerciser, the most important minerals influence muscular action and oxygen consumption. The muscle-related elements are calcium, phosphorus, sodium, potassium, and magnesium. Iron regulates the oxygen-transport system. Many foods contain these minerals, and supplemental capsules are aggressively marketed.

5. *Vitamins.* The ones that interest an active person most are E (which influences heart action and endurance), C (builds resistance and speeds healing) and the B-complex (promotes energy metabolism). As with minerals, vitamin requirements can be filled with foods, but commercial supplements also are readily available.

6. *Water.* Since the body is mostly water, you need a considerable fresh supply each day just to maintain essential fluid balance and to carry on normal bodily functions. With water, unlike food, there is little danger of taking too much. Excess food is stored as fat, and certain supplements (Vitamins A and D, for instance) can be taken in toxic amounts. The body simply flushes out excess water.

Following the U.S. government's Recommended Daily Allowances (RDAs) for these nutrients to the letter and number would require a computer. However, there's a simpler way to do it without counting every gram, milligram, and international unit.

The simplified method is the Basic Four that children learn in school. By following these guidelines, you fill most of the dietary requirements.

The Basic Four chart, based on traditional American eating habits, groups foods as follows:

- *Meat Group.* Two or three 3-ounce daily servings. Eggs, cheese, beans, or nuts may be substituted.
- *Milk Group.* Two or more glasses a day for adults. Cheese and similar milk-based products may supply part of this quota.
- *Vegetable/Fruit Group.* Four or more half-cup servings each day. Examples: dark green or deep yellow vegetables, citrus fruits.
- *Bread/Cereal Group.* Four or more servings, preferably whole grains.

Fats, sweets, and flavorings may be added. However, it is preferable to fill most of the caloric needs from the Basic Four.

These four—along with plenty of drinking water—provide every essential nutrient. If you eat these nutrients regularly, in proper amounts, and prepare them properly, there is no need for anything more. Manufactured vitamin and mineral supplements offer nothing that isn't available naturally in foods, and food is the more pleasant way than pills to take your nutrition.

Of course, the choices you make within these groupings also influence fitness. Increase your consumption of the healthful items listed in Table 8.1, while decreasing the quantities of less wholesome foods and drinks.

The American Heart Association recommends limiting the consumption of fat (to 30 percent of total calories), cholesterol (to no more than the amount found in one egg a day), salt (to less than 1 teaspoon daily) and alcohol (to the equivalent of two beers or less each day).

At the same time, seek out more fruits and vegetables (including juices), whole grains and other unrefined (complex) carbohydrates, and water.

Table 8.1
More or Less

Your goal: Establish new habits that will become permanent. The means to this end: Gradually modify your present habits instead of practicing extreme self-denial. Rather than trying to eat and drink only the "good" and eliminating all the "bad" immediately (and probably failing, then sliding back into old habits), concentrate on taking more of the former and less of the latter from the lists that follow.

Use more. . .	Use less. . .
Vegetable/fish/fowl proteins	Beef/pork/lamb meats
Vegetable oils	Animal fats (butter, lard)
Low-fat or skim milk	Whole milk/cream products
Whole-grain breads/cereals	White-flour products
Fresh fruits	Fatty, sugary desserts
Fresh vegetables	Canned vegetables
Herb flavorings, lemon juice	Salt in cooking/salt shaker
Decaffeinated coffee/tea	Caffeine drinks
Fruit and vegetable juices	Alcohol drinks
Plain water	Soda pop

Thought for the Day: How well do you balance your daily diet, and how can you improve it?

LESSON 30
The Athlete

Task for the Day: Learn the few special needs of the active person?

You hear contradictory dietary tales and end up wondering what to believe. At one extreme, athletes say they couldn't keep training without their organic, unadulterated diets. At the other, Olympians report living on pizza and beer. Diets of successful athletes vary so widely—from vegetarian to Vitamin J (for junk food)—that you might conclude it doesn't really make any difference what they eat.

If diets are judged by the performance results they give, "acceptable" eating obviously isn't limited to a few bland items. Exercisers can work well on a wide variety of fuels, and no one has yet determined a "best" diet for everyone all the time. "Normal" nutrition covers an extremely wide range of eating and drinking possibilities. Hundreds of combinations of nutrients can satisfy our wants and needs.

However, certain dietary adjustments do produce direct, measurable, and sometimes dramatic effects on physical endurance. A few may involve adding items, but more often you improve by taking something away.

You are what you eat—but as an aerobic exerciser you also very often are what you *don't* eat. That second axiom carries immediate and long-term implications.

Eating too much of the wrong items too soon before you exercise has uncomfortable consequences, ranging from cramps and nausea to vomiting. The old admonition not to swim for at least an hour after eating also applies to other activities.

The big problem in fitness-related nutrition is not deficiency but over-abundance. The long-term result of overeating is, of course, excessive weight—or more specifically, excessive *fat*. Most adults carry too much of it.

Each pound above ideal (and "ideal," as the Week 10 chapter explains, may be either more or less than the figure shown for you on standard weight tables) is an extra burden to carry. It creates a drag on mechanical and aerobic efficiency. The quickest way to improve performance, then, may be to shed a few pounds.

Weight is one of the most sensitive indicators of fitness, and all exercisers—whether overweight or not—should check theirs regularly. One of your three basic tools—along with training shoes and a watch for timing activity periods—is an accurate set of scales.

Regular physical activity tends to reduce weight, but not by dramatic amounts. Only exercise *plus* dieting can do that as quickly as most people want to slim down. Sudden losses or chronic underweight must be taken just as seriously. A quick drop often signals trouble from overwork, dehydration, or even true disease. Difficulty maintaining ideal weight can be a symptom of dietary inadequacy or even a serious medical condition.

The main item that most exercisers need more of is water. Runners, says the exercise physiologist who has studied this group most extensively, often become "chronically dehydrated." Dr. David Costill of Ball State University has found that athletes in training tend not to make up deficits from day to day and may have to remind themselves to take extra liquids.

Certain types of food intake—for instance, increased amounts of unrefined, so-called "complex" carbohydrates—do offer hope for eventual improvement in physical performance capacity. But don't expect miracles. Food and drink aren't ends but beginnings. Good nutrition is a catalyst that makes activity possible, but it offers no substitute for training and no shortcut to success. No exerciser ever simply ate and drank his or her way to success.

Treat your diet as neither a miracle-worker nor an enemy of fitness. Eating and drinking rate among life's great joys. As with training, you enjoy meals most when you've found the dietary balance between too little and too much.

Earlier in the book (Week 5), you were introduced to the idea that aerobic activity acts as a catalyst for adopting healthful habits: weight loss, more wholesome eating, and less smoking and alcohol drinking. Let's now examine those claims.

Runner's World magazine surveyed about 1,000 of its readers on these issues in 1979, with the following results. See where you fit, or would like to fit, into this profile:

WEIGHT

How effective is running as a weight-reducer? Amazing claims have been made for it, but what are the experiences of long-term runners?

This survey looked only at those who'd started as adults, since those who began as children would have shown weight gains unrelated to running. From this sample, two in every three lost weight, while the other one usually showed only slight gain or no change. Of the losers, 29 percent lost more than twenty pounds, while another 36 percent shed that amount or less.

One way to reduce weight is to take periodic fasts, eating nothing at all and drinking nothing stronger than juice. However, only 13 percent of *Runner's World* readers ever fast for 24 hours or longer. The majority apparently don't want to sacrifice the energy and pleasure that comes from regular eating.

SUPPLEMENTS

Medical opinion generally holds that heavy intake of supplements ranks some-where between useless and dangerous. Yet in this survey, 46 percent of run-ners said they take extra vitamins, the most popular being E and C. Activity reportedly drains away great amounts of magnesium and potassium, but almost no one in this group takes these minerals in capsule form.

Some commercial drinks, designed with the active person in mind, claim to replace the elements lost in sweat. Twenty-eight percent of the surveyed runners regularly take these drinks before, after, or during training.

SMOKING AND DRINKING

Less than 1 percent of these runners now smoke. But one in five of them had smoked regularly before starting to run. The running seems to have some effect, perhaps simply motivational but possibly physical as well, in weaning people from tobacco. While most runners abstain from smoking, about two-thirds of them take a drink now and then (and usually in moderate amounts). Beer and wine are favored over the harder liquors.

Thought for the Day: What can you do to change your habits, and what can the changes do for you?

LESSON 31
The Drinks

Task for the Day: Be sure you are getting enough to drink.

During exercise, you sweat off weight much faster than you burn it off. Calories only burn at the rate of about 100 for each mile run or walked. At this rate, you must train two or three weeks to lose a pound of flesh. On the other hand, a pound of fluid may drain away in two or three miles. On hot days, sweat pours out even faster. (Don't interpret this as a shortcut weight-reduction gim-mick. You've lost *sweat,* but only temporarily, and nothing has happened to your true weight.)

While fluid losses are temporary, they're still vitally important to exer-cisers. The significant effects are negative, ranging from impaired perfor-mance to heat collapse. Here is what happens: A pint of sweat weighs about one pound, and an exerciser can lose a quart or so before noticing anything is wrong. As the deficit grows, the body temperature rises proportionately—pushing toward a critical level.

Table 8.2
Sweat Debt

Fluid losses exceeding 3 percent of body weight represent significant dehydration. This table translates the 3 percent figures into pounds for exercisers of various sizes. Check your pre- and post-activity weight in hot, humid weather. To get the most accurate reading of your sweat debt, weigh immediately after training—and before drinking.

Before	After	Before	After
100 pounds	97	155 pounds	150
105 pounds	102	160 pounds	155
110 pounds	107	165 pounds	160
115 pounds	112	170 pounds	165
120 pounds	116	175 pounds	170
125 pounds	121	180 pounds	175
130 pounds	126	185 pounds	180
135 pounds	131	190 pounds	184
140 pounds	136	195 pounds	189
145 pounds	141	200 pounds	194
150 pounds	145	205 pounds	199

C. H. Wyndham, a South African, has done extensive research on heat responses. He says, "Up to a water deficit of about 3 percent, body temperature varies between about 101 and 102 degrees. But with an increase in water deficit above 3 percent, rectal temperatures increase in proportion to the extent of water deficit." (Find your 3-percent warning level in Table 8.2.)

The 2- or 3-degree temperature rise is normal and acceptable during vigorous activity. But increases beyond that point bear watching. Physiologist Dr. David Costill has measured sweat losses as great as 10 percent in marathon runners, and temperatures as high as 105 degrees.

A reading only slightly higher than that figure can lead to heat exhaustion or heat stroke, the latter being potentialy fatal. But don't be alarmed. You're unlikely to overheat during comfortably paced training lasting less than an hour.

Drinking immediately before, during, and after exercise sessions won't completely eliminate losses. But it can replace enough of the lost fluid and cool temperatures to a degree where activity is at least safe.

Dr. Costill says athletes tend to let the sensation of thirst set their drinking habits, and thirst sometimes fibs about true fluid needs. "In laboratory tests that required about 8 pounds of sweat loss," he says, "we found that thirst was temporarily satisfied by drinking as little as 1 pound of water." (Water accounts for nearly all of the loss, and is the replacement drink of choice because it is asorbed quickest and with fewest complications.)

After a large sweat loss, it may take a day or more to redress the balance. Chronic dehydration may result from repeated heavy drains and inadequate replacement. The best way to guard against this condition is to check your weight each day. If you're still down more than 2 pounds from the day before, you're a quart low on liquids. Drink up!

Thought for the Day: *How much weight do you typically lose during a hot-weather training session?*

LESSON 32
The Extras

Task for the Day: *Assess your needs for vitamin/mineral supplements.*

Dr. Ludvig Prokop is not a food faddist. The Austrian is one of the world's most respected sports physicians. His stand in the great supplements-for-athletes debate is that they may improve performance. But he carefully qualifies his statements. Dr. Prokop cautions that vitamins produce only "a demonstrable and subjectively noticeable influence on performance when errors are made in composition and amounts in the diet. With full-valued diet, if one adds even high amounts of vitamins, he can expect little positive effect."

Prokop's position is one commonly held among doctors and dieticians: Added amounts of vitamins and minerals, beyond supplies in the normal diet, improve exercise performance only if they correct deficiencies. If no deficits exist, nothing good happens. Money spent on supplements is therefore wasted.

The debate, then, centers on deficiencies. How common are they? And are they likely to occur in exercisers more than in non-exercisers? Some experts feel that the Recommended Daily Allowances (RDAs) drawn up by the Nutritional Board of the National Academy of Sciences are more than satisfactory, and that the typical American diet provides all the nutrients required to stay healthy.

However, a U.S. Department of Agriculture survey found that two-thirds of the American population fell below the recommended level in at least one nutrient. A conservative diet expert would answer that the RDAs have built-in safety margins, and that most people can get along quite well on less than the recommended amounts. Ludvig Prokop says a non-athlete may be able to do this, but not an active person. He notes, "In hard work, the need for various vitamins increases markedly, so that even with so-called 'normal' doses a deficiency can result."

Deficiencies in Vitamins C and E are common according to Dr. Prokop. The American recommendations are 60 milligrams of C and 30 international units of E daily per grown men (slightly less for women). For endurance athletes, Dr. Prokop would triple or quadruple the Vitamin C intake (to between 200 to 240 milligrams), and would nearly double the Vitamin E level (to no more than 50 international units). Both vitamins influence endurance and recovery powers.

However, Prokop warns again that these increased doses are used only to make up for deficiencies. Overdoses, he says, "can easily disturb the balance and thereby *decrease* performance capacity." (And with some supplements, excessive amounts can be toxic.)

That leads to another side of the argument over supplements: What constitutes an "overdose"? Dr. Gabe Mirkin, a well-known American author on sports medicine, tells of an experience he once had. "I would take 500 milligrams of Vitamin C twice a day. I noted that whenever I stopped taking it, my recovery periods from long runs was prolonged and my mileage would go down. I even wrote in a newspaper article that Vitamin C appeared to improve my endurance."

Then Dr. Mirkin was injured. He quit taking his C. When he recovered, he found that he no longer needed the vitamin pills. His workouts were as good as before. "I attributed my early dependence to the fact that when I took large doses of Vitamin C, my body *required* large doses," he says.

The lesson here is: If you think you need suplements, take small amounts. They're cheaper that way, if not safer.

Thought for the Day: *Do you take vitamin supplements to fortify your body or to ease your mind?*

Now turn to Table 8.3 to log in your training time for the week.

Table 8.3
Week 8 Training Chart

Record your physical training for the week, including only formal sessions, not incidental daily exercise. List the actual date, aerobic activity, duration in minutes, and any supplemental "muscle" exercises. A suggested weekly program would include four aerobic training days, lasting at least 30 minutes, with not more than two training days in a row or more than two straight rest days.

Day (Date)	Aerobic Exercise	Duration	Other Exercise
Sunday			
Monday			
Tuesday			
Wednesday			
Thursday			
Friday			
Saturday			

Total aerobic training time for the week: _____

Number of aerobic sessions: _____

Average time per session: _____

WEEK 9

Diet Changes

LESSON 33
The Hunger

Task for the Day: Introduce yourself to the dietary theories and practices of George Sheehan.

Dr. Sheehan once called himself a "dietary agnostic." He said that arguing with an athlete or exerciser about diet is "like debating a true believer on religion." Both subjects offer lots of room for interpretation and opinion, and few absolute answers.

For many years after launching his running and sports medicine careers in the 1960s, Sheehan paid little attention to dietary matters. For instance, he tells of one exchange after a lecture. The first question was about diet.

"Well, I don't have much to say about it," Sheehan answered.

The man asking the question persisted. He reminded the doctor that he had been advertised as saying a few words about diet.

"I just have," said Sheehan. "Next question. . ."

But the subject wouldn't go away that easily. So his thinking and writing and speaking about it have increased. While he hasn't become a true believer, he has softened his previous agnosticism.

Dr. Sheehan illustrates another story. The party line in his profession is that vitamin supplements are unnecessary. Doctors generally say that vitamins taken in amounts greater than required, and obtained naturally from foods, are flushed out as "expensive urine."

Sheehan recalls hearing a speaker at a medical convention. The man asked during his talk, "How many of you recommend supplemental vitamins to your patients?" Only a few hands went up. The doctors who put them up looked embarrassed at being caught violating the party line.

"Okay," the speaker said, "now I want to know how many of *you* take extra vitamins." Hands went up throughout the audience. People laughed as they looked around and saw the number of confessions being made.

"Just as I thought," said the man onstage. After admitting that he too gulped down a handful of pills each day, he told his colleagues, "We are like atheists who still go to church each Sunday—just in case we might be wrong in our nonbelief."

George Sheehan himself has adopted progressively better dietary habits over the years—just to be sure he hasn't missed something. The subject has taken an increasingly prominent place in his writing and speaking.

We devote this week's lessons largely to Dr. Sheehan's advice on diet-related matters. He offers a refreshing mixture of belief and skepticism on this topic too often weighted down with dogma. For instance, the abuses of sugars and fats have given them bad names in the medical, dental, nutritional, and fitness communities. Sheehan has kinder words for these substances than do many of his colleagues, who often make sugar and fat sound like poison.

Good storyteller that he is, Dr. Sheehan leads into this subject with an ancedote: "When noted running researcher Dr. David Costill did a physiological profile on marathoner Bill Rodgers, he learned something about Rodgers' eating habits." He didn't learn it from a scientific test but from simple observation. "Costill was eating lunch in the laboratory when Rodgers arrived, so Dave invited him to sit down for some preliminary discussion," says Sheehan.

Rodgers, normally the best of talkers, seemed preoccupied. Instead of looking at Costill, he stared at the physiologist's dessert. Realizing that his research was going nowhere as long as they had this barrier between them, Costill finally said, "Would you like this piece of pie, Bill?"

It was eaten almost before the doctor had finished his question. Rodger's appetite and food preferences are almost as legendary as his running ability.

George Sheehan says, "Like many high-mileage runners, he will eat almost anything. But he leans toward cake and pie, candy and pastry, soft drinks, and beer."

While Sheehan the doctor would prefer that carbohydrate needs be filled mostly from more natural, "complex" sources, Sheehan the athlete knows the appetites of a person in training. "Apparently, this is the diet that runners' instincts tell them is best. As their mileage increases, so does their need for quick-energy 'junk food.' "

He says that vigorous exercise "affects the 'appestat.' This is the instinct which tells us what, when and how much to eat. The thermostat-like system shuts down when we sit around too much, but exercise keeps it working."

Our cravings for sugar and starch are signs that the appestat is working. Bill Rodgers runs 120 or more miles a week, and at less than 130 pounds he doesn't have a very large fuel tank. To keep his energy up, his appestat tells him to take a 2 A.M. snack of milk and cookies to power his morning run.

Sheehan lists his own top two dietary rules: "First, I must carry the least weight possible. Second, I must have the most available energy possible." He says, "The first must be accomplished without losing strength, the second without gaining weight." This would be a hard line to walk if it were not for the automatic appestat telling us what, when, and how much to eat.

Fat has long been portrayed as the enemy of the fit. This has been accepted as true both for fat worn on the body as excess baggage and fat taken in as food. So exercisers have leaned toward lightness in what they eat and what they carry. They've sometimes leaned too far.

Dr. Sheehan favors leanness but warns against extreme skinniness. He reports a study of ballet dancers who trained 6 to 8 hours a day—far more than an aerobic exerciser would. Their casualty rate from bone, muscle, and tendon injuries was high. The researchers found that the dancers most prone to injuries were those on diets that held them below 2,000 calories a day. The healthiest were those who ate what their appetites requested.

The exercising body demands its prime energy sources—lots of carbohydrates and small but regular amounts of fat. These foodstuffs are the very same ones a dieter tries to eliminate first as "too fattening," and are the first to be missed.

Thought for the Day: *Are you arbitrarily depriving yourself of items your body needs?*

LESSON 34
The Upsets

Task for the Day: *Find the causes of digestive problems during exercise.*

It's said you don't miss the water until the well runs dry. You also don't appreciate how important proper nutrition is until something goes wrong inside. If you're eating correctly, you ignore your internal workings. But when those organs scream for relief, you must pay attention.

Exercisers choose to operate under physical stress and strain. This temporarily stressful situation makes them particularly susceptible to diet-related irregularities that don't often strike people who operate on a lower plane.

There are two main causes of internal distress:

■ *Eating too much, too close to exercise time.* We train best on an empty or nearly empty stomach.

Arthur Lydiard, a prominent running coach from New Zealand, observes that he rarely sees athletes "collapse from malnutrition" while training or competing. But they frequently have problems of the opposite type: doubling over with side pains called "stitches," making "pitstops" during a run, or having an unpleasant sloshing and bloated feeling.

Sugared foods and drinks can also play tricks on you. Dr. George Sheehan recalls once taking a sweet drink about an hour before training and almost fainting during the run. What had occurred, he knows now, was "reactive hypoglycemia." The drink had triggered a quick rise in his blood sugar. The sugar level had peaked during the hour's wait, then had plunged before the run started.

Eat lightly, if at all, in the last few hours before exercising. Your body holds abundant stored energy to carry you through the activity. If you drink, make it water.

The one basic rule in both the timing and type of that pre-activity meal: Err on the side of too little rather than too much. When in doubt about an item, don't eat or drink it.

■ *Eating the wrong foods at the wrong times.* Some people can't tolerate certain food groups, and react violently to them—particularly in times of stress.

Surprisingly, two chief culprits may be the "perfect food" and the "staff of life." Dr. Sheehan notes that a great number of pleas for help come from athletes and exercisers who don't tolerate milk and bread products very well.

Dr. Sheehan identifies other suspect foods as: the highly allergenic ones (for example, chocolate, shellfish, strawberries, pork, melon, nuts, citrus fruits, egg whites) and those high in fiber (raw fruits and vegetables, whole grains, nuts, corn, beans). According to Sheehan, these foods may "cause stomach pains, diarrhea, bloating, rash, itching, headaches, nasal stuffiness, etc."

The irony, Sheehan points out, is that bread and milk—long considered the perfect foods for stomach disorders—have turned out to be a leading cause of the ailments in exercisers and athletes. He describes symptoms from one of his patients, a long-distance runner named Gary.

"Every time he had a tough race or workout," says Sheehan, "he came down with severe stomach pains. Sometimes he would have diarrhea and blood [in his stools] as well. When not running and at all other times, he had little or no bowel complaints."

When Gary first sought help from a different doctor, he was told nothing was abnormal and that his difficulties stemmed from "too much stress during a race and too much nervousness anticipating it." Gary already knew that. But telling a distance runner to avoid stress is like telling a swimmer not to get wet.

"Stress obviously played a part," Sheehan continue͏
oped symptoms after a hard run. But he was peculiarly s͏
abdominal complaints, and no one knew why. He had no k͏
even varying his pre-run meal didn't help. He continued͏
severe enough to double him up after the run. He finally͏
bread and milk, but he still had trouble. There, as it turne͏

Gluten, a protein found in all grains except corn and rice, w͏
problem. "Many of us, when put under stress, can become symptomatic,"
explains Dr. Sheehan. "Gluten is always there in our diet—in the bread and
baked goods, in the cereals and cereal products, and hidden in soups and
gravies, ice cream, wheat germ, mayonnaise, and even beer and ale."

This athlete suffered from a food intolerance, which Sheehan defines
as "the inability to eat certain foods without the likelihood of some reaction
or malfunction. Food intolerance is a much wider concept than food allergy.
It includes, in addition to the usual allergic hypersensitivity, many other mech-
anisms—some unknown—by which food can cause body reactions."

He advises, "If you have symptoms presumably due to nerves or stress
or hypoglycemia, or if your arthritis or migraine or other chronic disease seems
worse than it should be, think 'food intolerance.' Learn the true cause of your
complaints." This can be done by adding or excluding suspect items, and by
noting the reactions in a food diary. "Some foods are seldom eaten, but when
consumed cause violent symptoms," says Dr. Sheehan. "Common examples
are lobster, crab, chocolate, and seasonal fruits." With athletes and exercisers, however, "the problem most often rises from staples like milk, eggs,
wheat, coffee, or tea. Almost always, the source is consumed daily."

He views formal allergy testing by doctors for these complaints as unnecessary and often inconclusive. Sheehan prefers "intelligent trial and error—
the exclusion diet." This method relies on the subtraction and addition of various foods in an attempt to find one or more causes of the trouble. "One
method is to limit intake for one week to a single meat, a single fruit, and
water. If symptoms are relieved, one food is reintroduced each week to see
what specific food provokes symptoms. Simpler is to go with the statistics,
and exclude milk, milk products, eggs, and wheat. If that diet fails to relieve
symptoms, another three of the more commonly implicated foods can be re-
moved the following week."

When the culprit is an item seldom eaten, the detective work is even
easier. "A food diary will pinpoint the food taken before each episode," says
Dr. Sheehan. "Your body will have given the answer."

Thought for the Day: *Are you eating or drinking things that you
like but that* don't *like you?*

LESSON 35
The Smoking

Task for the Day: *Learn about one of the most dangerous and habit-forming drugs—nicotine.*

Dr. George Sheehan takes a surprisingly soft line on smoking. Not that he has ever smoked or would recommend it to anyone else. He knows full well that tobacco smoke is a leading cause of the illnesses that he, as a physician, must treat. Yet Dr. Sheehan also appreciates the hold that smoking has on people. "In some of my patients, the satisfactions received from smoking seemed worth the statistical dangers," he says. "There were certain instances where the actual and immediate complications attending withdrawal outweighed the theoretical benefits in the future."

Stopping smoking isn't usually as simple as wanting to quit, although some people do give up cigarettes cold turkey. Sheehan notes that "in some individuals, no threat of future disease is effective. They will continue even after the [smoking-related] diseases arrive and take their toll." For instance, "Emphysema patients are inclined to keep smoking. They are unable to stop a practice that contributed to their present state and is aggravating it further. Almost as unbelievable is the continued smoking by a patient after a heart attack or coronary surgery."

Why? Simply stated, smoking is habit-forming. The smoker can become addicted.

"The drug that makes this happen is nicotine," says Dr. Sheehan. "It provides arousal for necessary tasks, then produces the calm and relaxation wanted when the tasks are over. Stopping smoking results in psychological distress, the loss of arousal on the one hand and the loss of relaxation on the other."

He adds that "withdrawal from this habit is attended by psychological symptoms. No one would minimize them. Withdrawal from addiction adds physiological disturbances worse than many disease states, and nicotine is one of the most powerful addictive substances known. Smoking-cessation programs have failure rates that almost exactly match those seen in heroin programs. At the end of a year, only about one-quarter of the patients in antismoking therapies have achieved abstinence."

George Sheehan recommends not giving up anything "until you don't need it any more." He says, "The task is not only to abstain and to fight the symptoms brought on by abstinence. We must find a substitute that will restore our normal function." Not surprisingly, he prefers aerobic exercise.

Dr. Sheehan considers withdrawal programs and techniques as essential "first aid" against smoking. However, "The long term must be total retraining of the person who was a smoker."

Thought for the Day: Do you smoke—and if so, when and how do you plan to stop?

LESSON 36
The Alcohol

Task for the Day: See how athletes and exercisers handle this most common of "recreational" drugs.

Unlike tobacco, alcohol falls into a gray area where its use is neither recommended nor condemned for active people. Athletes and exercisers do drink it, and without apparent ill effects provided they stay within their limits.

Dr. George Sheehan's association with this substance has, by his own admission, "taken several twists and turns during my life"—from near-total abstinence as a young athlete to overindulgence as a middle-aged and sedentary doctor.

"I rarely touched alcohol while I was running in college," he says. "I preferred a half-pint of vanilla ice cream to my fellow students' couple or three beers. Then came private medical practice, with those rare days off—and with them, fancy drinking bouts."

He recalls that "my alcohol intake went down to almost zero when I began running at age 45. I felt no need for a relaxant or a confidence booster or something to produce an altered state of consciousness. Running did all that."

Dr. Sheehan later chose the moderate path between these extremes. "Now, with my practice past, and the running a part of a bigger pattern of writing and lecturing and traveling, I find those two beers at night something I look forward to. They are a fine way to end the day."

Having said this, he goes on to label alcohol "a loaded gun. It must be handled carefully. More than a hundred diseases have been attributed to alcohol abuse. Alcohol doesn't need anyone to give it a bad name. It already has one."

Still, it is a fact of life and is likely to remain so. "It permeates our whole culture," says Sheehan. "The discussion of its use has been going on since the dawn of civilization. Alcohol in some form has always been part of celebrations and festivals and carnivals—at events that are larger than life."

Or maybe it just makes these events appear that way. According to this doctor, "The main reason we use alcohol is to alter our consciousness. That alteration may be extremely minor, simply making us perceive this party we are attending as interesting and entertaining. It may be as major as having a peak experience."

Sheehan then identifies the problem: "If only we could hew to the line, and stop when we have achieved sociability and insight and a new feeling about life."

He typically stops at two beers (the alcohol-equivalent that is the American Heart Association's recommended daily limit). They are the end of his working day, his celebration of it.

"I can do nothing creative after two beers," says Sheehan. "So when I finally sit down and open up a beer, it is the signal that the day is over. This is the seal. I am ready to put this present twenty-four hours into the history books and get ready for a new tomorrow."

Thought for the Day: *Can you stop with the second beer?*

Now turn to Table 9.1 to log in your training time for the week.

Table 9.1
Week 9 Training Chart

Record your physical training for the week, including only formal sessions, not incidental daily exercise. List the actual date, aerobic activity, duration in minutes, and any supplemental "muscle" exercises. A suggested weekly program would include four aerobic training days, lasting at least 30 minutes, with not more than two training days in a row or more than two straight rest days.

Day (Date)	Aerobic Exercise	Duration	Other Exercise
Sunday			
Monday			
Tuesday			
Wednesday			
Thursday			
Friday			
Saturday			

Total aerobic training time for the week: _____

Number of aerobic sessions: _____

Average time per session: _____

WEEK
10

Weight
Control

LESSON 37
The Fat

Task for the Day: Determine how much you should weigh.

Calories measure total food intake. Scientifically speaking, a calorie (technically a "kilocalorie" but generally known by its shorter name) is the amount of heat required to raise the temperature of 1 kilogram of water 1 degree centigrade. Nutritionally speaking, calories are the units you must take in and save to gain weight, or avoid and spend to lose it. A pound of body weight contains about 3,500 calories of energy. To gain 1 pound, you must consume and store that much. To lose 1 pound, the reverse is true; you have to get rid of the stored weight.

All activities burn calories. Even sitting in a rocking chair, reading the newspaper, uses them at the rate of about a quarter of a calorie per pound per hour. Moderate exercise, such as working in the garden, increases the rate to about a half-calorie. During vigorous walking, the expenditure jumps to 2 or 3 calories per minute. On the run, that amount doubles.

All carbohydrate, fat, and protein foods contain calories. Water, minerals, and vitamins do not. For moderately active adults, the recommended caloric intake is 16 to 18 per pound per day. This totals 2,400 to 2,700 for a 150-pound man, and 1,900 to 2,200 for a 120-pound woman.

Obviously, daily caloric intake can't be reduced to a formula that applies to everyone. You have to make yourself what Dr. George Sheehan calls an "experiment of one." Determine your own needs. Weight is the most accessible guide. Decide the weight at which you might look and feel and exercise best, and then try to work down or up to that figure. It's as simple as balancing calories consumed with calories spent. It's simple *on paper,* that is. In practice, this isn't so easy—either to pinpoint ideal weight or to achieve it.

One method is to labor through a trial-and-error process, measuring weight against physical performance. This can take years. Another way is to consult a standard weight chart. This almost invariably lets you weigh either too much or too little. Or you can use simplistic rules of thumb that don't take into account the differences in frame sizes. These apply to people of average build.

The most reliable measure of proper weight for your frame is a check of body composition. This determines your fat percentage. "Ideals," regardless of how chunky or lean an individual might look or what the scales might say, generally are listed as 12 to 15 percent for men, and 18 to 22 percent for women.

This technique involves measurements with calipers or weighing in a water tank. These tests aren't as readily available as the bathroom scales, but are important enough to seek out.

As your next best guidelines, use weight to estimate fat. Have the percentage checked by a professional, then establish your lean body weight from this figure.

Lean weight is a skin-and-bones reading: what you would be at zero-percent fat. If your tester doesn't tell you that number, you can calculate it quickly by multiplying your current weight by the "lean" percentage. For example, you weigh 150 pounds. A body fat reading of 15 percent means 85 percent is lean mass. 150 times .85 equals a lean weight of 127.5 pounds.

Once you have this baseline figure, weigh yourself regularly and use Table 10.1 to find your body fat reading at any one time. Remember that the target ranges are 18 to 22 percent for women, and 12 to 15 percent for men.

Table 10.1
Weight/Fat Readings

Read down the left column of the table to find the figure closest to your lean weight. (It won't change dramatically once you've settled into an exercise program. What fluctuates is the fat percentage.)

Move across the page on that line to the figure nearest your current true weight. (Note that the table comes in three parts with fat ranges of 10 to 15 percent, 16 to 21, and 22 to 27.)

Look to the top of that column for your approximate present body fat reading. (Have your body fat retested once or twice a year to establish current lean weight.)

Body Fat Percentages 10-15

Lean Weight	10%	11%	12%	13%	14%	15%
90 pounds	100	101	102	103	105	106
95 pounds	106	107	108	109	111	112
100 pounds	111	112	114	115	116	118
105 pounds	117	118	120	122	123	124
110 pounds	122	123	125	127	128	130
115 pounds	128	129	131	133	134	136
120 pounds	133	134	136	138	139	141
125 pounds	139	140	142	144	145	147
130 pounds	144	146	148	150	151	153
135 pounds	150	152	154	156	157	159
140 pounds	155	157	159	161	163	165
145 pounds	161	163	165	167	169	171
150 pounds	166	168	171	173	175	177
155 pounds	172	174	177	179	181	183
160 pounds	178	180	182	184	186	188
165 pounds	184	186	188	190	192	194
170 pounds	189	191	193	195	197	200
175 pounds	195	197	199	201	203	206
180 pounds	200	202	205	207	209	212

Table 10.1—*Continued*

Body Fat Percentages 16–21

Lean Weight	16%	17%	18%	19%	20%	21%
90 pounds	107	109	110	111	112	114
95 pounds	113	115	116	118	119	121
100 pounds	119	120	122	124	125	127
105 pounds	125	126	128	130	132	134
110 pounds	131	132	134	136	138	140
115 pounds	137	138	140	142	144	146
120 pounds	143	144	146	148	150	152
125 pounds	149	151	153	155	157	158
130 pounds	155	157	159	161	163	165
135 pounds	161	163	165	167	169	171
140 pounds	167	169	171	173	175	177
145 pounds	173	175	177	180	182	184
150 pounds	179	181	183	186	188	190
155 pounds	185	187	189	192	194	196
160 pounds	191	193	195	198	200	202
165 pounds	197	199	201	204	207	209
170 pounds	203	205	207	210	213	215
175 pounds	209	211	213	216	219	222
180 pounds	214	216	219	222	225	228

Table 10.1—Continued

Body Fat Percentages 22–27

Lean Weight	22%	23%	24%	25%	26%	27%
90 pounds	115	117	118	120	122	124
95 pounds	121	124	125	127	129	131
100 pounds	129	130	132	134	136	137
105 pounds	136	137	138	141	143	144
110 pounds	142	143	145	147	150	151
115 pounds	148	150	152	154	157	158
120 pounds	154	156	158	161	163	165
125 pounds	161	163	165	168	170	172
130 pounds	167	169	172	174	176	178
135 pounds	174	176	179	181	183	185
140 pounds	179	182	185	187	190	192
145 pounds	186	189	192	194	197	199
150 pounds	193	195	198	201	204	206
155 pounds	200	202	205	208	211	213
160 pounds	206	208	211	214	217	220
165 pounds	213	215	218	221	224	227
170 pounds	219	221	224	227	230	233
175 pounds	225	228	231	234	237	240
180 pounds	231	234	237	241	244	247

Thought for the Day: Do you know exactly how fat you are today?

LESSON 38
The Scales

Task for the Day: Learn the value of a daily weigh-in.

Weight-watching is the great American pastime. Everyone talks about weight, but rarely is much done to change it. However, exercisers can't afford just to talk about theirs, because weight is critical to them. If it slips outside the narrow boundaries of the ideal range, performance shows it. You have to establish weight where you think it belongs, then ensure that it stays there. For this reason, your scales are as important to you as your shoes and watch. A daily weight record is as valuable as a daily exercise log.

Keep the following weight-watching pointers in mind. Some are suggestions, others warnings:

1. *Decide on ideal weight.* Start by having your body fat checked, and use your weight to keep tabs on that percentage (see Table 10.1). Then observe at what fat level you look, feel, and perform best.

2. *Reach that ideal weight.* If you're not there already, chances are you're on the high side. There are lots of ways to reduce—all of which involve (a) work, (b) sacrifice, or (c) both—exercising and dieting, in other words.

3. *Lose gradually.* The only successful diets are those that modify overall eating habits and are fairly easy to maintain for periods of months and years. Drastic, quick-loss schemes are often self-defeating because they're hard to stick with, and may disrupt internal equilibrium or drag down performance.

4. *Keep a record.* Weigh every day at the same time and under the same conditions. An easy system to follow is weighing yourself first thing each morning, after you've gone to the bathroom and before you've put on clothes, exercised, or had breakfast. Write the weight alongside the record of daily activity (such as in Table 10.3).

5. *Don't be fooled by false losses.* These are fluid losses. An aerobic exerciser can easily lose several pounds a day. In a year's time, you may sweat away a half-ton of weight. Obviously, these are temporary losses, lasting only as long as it takes to do some heavy drinking. The liquid losses needn't concern you unless they show up the next morning in a 2- or 3-pound weight drop, which signal chronic dehydration.

6. *Watch for creeping gains.* Overnight gains are easy enough to handle; just eat lightly until you're back to normal. The hard ones to catch are those you hardly notice. A few extra calories a day may add no more than a few ounces a month, but over a year's time these ounces multiply into pounds. You wake up one morning five years later and realize you've gained 10 pounds. Here again, daily weight-watching prevents unpleasant surprises.

7. *Don't gorge.* Exercising isn't an invitation to gluttony. Running and walking consume about 100 calories per mile, and one good workout is worth only a few hundred. One extra dessert can more than cancel out those gains.

8. *Don't starve.* The weight and fat levels can fall too low to support activity and health. Treat sudden losses or a chronic underweight condition as seriously as you would treat being overweight.

Thought for the Day: *How much do you weigh today?*

LESSON 39
The Diet

Task for the Day: *Consider the odds against winning the battle against fat by dieting alone.*

Dr. George Sheehan spells out the options in blunt terms: "The overweight person is faced with three choices—be fat, be hungry, or exercise. If you weigh too much, you can stay where you are, go on a diet, or get moving." He then examines the three possibilities: "The first choice is unacceptable. Everyone would rather be lean and trim and slim. Yet by middle-age, more than 50 percent of Americans are overweight—and hating it."

Dr. Sheehan refers to the second choice as ineffective. "The war against fat will not be won by dieting." Extreme caloric restriction, he says, "is a delusion. It yields victories that almost invariably become defeats, and leads to losses that are nearly always regained. Food restriction may temporarily decrease weight, but this loss cannot be maintained."

Sheehan says the odds are stacked twenty-to-one against success in dieting. Yet "one-quarter of our adult population is dieting to lose weight. These people have accepted the alternative to being fat: being hungry. In order to maintain weight loss, they have to eat less and less. They must resign themselves to an unceasing craving for food."

The great majority lose this battle of the bulge. Dr. Sheehan notes that "most obese people do not remain in treatment. Of those who lose weight, most will regain it. Only about 3 percent of dieters lose weight and keep it off. Weight goes down but then goes up again in this unending battle. Fat retreats and is held at bay for a while, only to advance and once more rule the day."

If dieting isn't the answer, what is? The third alternative: exercise, by itself or in combination with a moderation of eating quantities. George Sheehan himself needed none of the latter when he started exercising aerobically.

"When I began running," he says, "I weighed 160 pounds. I was reasonably active at the time, and some people took me for an athlete. I played tennis when weather permitted, squash when it didn't. My 30 miles of running a week soon brought me down to 136 pounds, my weight when I ran in college. Tests showed I was 9 percent body fat, even though I made no conscious change in my diet then and none since."

Dr. Sheehan would reach a state dieters can only dream about. While in heavy training, he had to work at keeping his weight *up*.

Thought for the Day: *Do you choose to be heavy, hungry, or active?*

LESSON 40
The Exercise

Task for the Day: *See why obesity is more closely related to underworking than overeating.*

Dr. George Sheehan takes his cues on this subject from Covert Bailey, author of the best-selling book *Fit or Fat?* (Houghton Mifflin, 1977). Bailey maintains that people are not overweight; they are *overfat*. The goal, then, is less to lose weight than to trim fat without sacrificing functioning muscle tissue.

"Dieting alone will not do the job," says Dr. Sheehan. "Dieting reduces muscle as well as fat. It produces haggard people who do not look good or feel good. Covert Bailey is quick to point this out. He has little faith in dieting.

"Nor is Bailey impressed with pounds lost. When a person tells him that he or she has lost 12 pounds or more on a diet, he asks, '12 pounds of what?' Some of it is fat, of course. But some of it is water, which means nothing. And some of it is muscle, which means the dieter has actually lost ground rather than gained it."

Covert Bailey calls exercise the best cure for obesity. George Sheehan agrees, and adds, "This exercise should be aerobic and done at a comfortable level. It should involve as many muscle groups as possible, thereby emphasizing walking, running, bicycling, and swimming. Finally, it should last for 30 minutes to an hour and be done at least three times a week. Duration is more important than intensity. Obesity is conquered as we increase our muscle mass and increase the muscle enzymes that burn up the fats and carbohydrates we eat. The way to do this—the *only* way we can do it, Bailey maintains—is to exercise regularly."

As noted, weight itself doesn't concern Bailey. Fatness and fitness do. He observes that one person can weigh 250 pounds and have a fat reading in the "fit" range, while another can weigh half as much and be classified as obese.

Once you have achieved fitness, you may get to quit worrying about how much you eat. Dr. Sheehan says that "most fat people actually eat less than skinny people. The endurance athlete, a lean and active creature, is often an insatiable eater—yet gains no weight." These athletes "look upon food as their friend, while dieters look upon it as the enemy. While dieters are engaged in hand-to-hand combat against food, endurance athletes are eating to their hearts' content."

Physical activity does burn calories, but not as quickly as you might think or hope. The figure generally quoted for running and walking is 100 calories per mile. At that rate, you must cover 5 to 10 miles to work off that fast-food snack you ate last night. You must train 35 miles to drop a single pound, and that is assuming you don't increase your eating in response to the extra exercise.

If you plan to lose weight by exercising, accept the fact that you'll take it off slowly. Say you're running/walking 3 miles, five days a week, while keeping food intake constant. That effort equals about 1,500 calories weekly, so you can plan on losing a pound every two to three weeks. That may not sound like much. But in a year's time it can add up to 20 pounds—without dieting. With dietary limitations, the timetable can be speeded up.

On this note, a warning: Resist the temptation to indulge in quick-loss schemes. They usually lead to declines in energy and artificial water-weight losses. While dieting, you're tempted to cut out high-carbohydrate foods such as grains, potatoes, and sugars—the very items you need to sustain activity. Excessive sweating from training in rubberized or heavy clothing may take off several pounds, but it doesn't stay lost.

Think of weight reduction as a long-term project that will be permanent on completion.

Table 10.2
Caloric Costs

All foods and most drinks contain calories. Exercise consumes them. Activities vary in their effectiveness as fuel-burners, as the following table indicates. Listed are rough estimates of caloric consumption for the popular aerobic exercises during exercise periods of 30, 45, and 60 minutes. This information is taken from Dr. Peter Wood's *California Diet and Exercise Programs* (Anderson/World, 1983). Precise calorie use depends on your intensity of effort and level of fitness.

Note that a mile of either running or walking consumes about 100 calories, but it typically takes about twice as much time to walk a distance as it does to run it. To lose 1 pound without changing your diet, you must exercise away approximately 3,500 calories. This equals about 35 running/walking miles.

(Table 3.1 contains more details on the activities listed here.)

Activity	30 min.	45 min.	60 min.	1 pound
Running	300	450	600	6 hours
Bicycling	300	450	600	6 hours
Swimming	300	450	600	6 hours
X-C skiing	300	450	600	6 hours
Run/walk	225	335	450	8 hours
Aerobic dance	225	335	450	8 hours
Rowing	225	335	450	8 hours
Walking	150	225	300	12 hours
Active games	150	225	300	12 hours

Thought for the Day: *What was the caloric cost of your most recent training session?*

Now use Table 10.3 to log in your training time for the week.

Table 10.3
Week 10 Training Chart

Record your physical training for the week, including only formal sessions, not incidental daily exercise. List the actual date, aerobic activity, duration in minutes, and any supplemental "muscle" exercises. A suggested weekly program would include four aerobic training days, lasting at least 30 minutes, with not more than two training days in a row or more than two straight rest days.

Day (Date)	Aerobic Exercise	Duration	Other Exercise
Sunday			
Monday			
Tuesday			
Wednesday			
Thursday			
Friday			
Saturday			

Total aerobic training time for the week: _____

Number of aerobic sessions: _____

Average time per session: _____

PART
Four

Yourself

WEEK 11

Mind Training

LESSON 41
The Symptoms

Task for the Day: Introduce yourself to the concept that exercise is much more than a physical act.

"Years ago," write walking promoters Aaron Sussman and Ruth Goode, "scientists were predicting the evolution of [humans] without legs, thanks to the automobile. Nowadays, we know they were wrong. It is not our legs we are losing. It is our minds."

Movement, self-propelled movement, is strong medicine. With it, we promote physical health. Without it, we deteriorate. We know that. Less obvious is the effect movement has on mental health. The head apparently requires this kind of exercise just as much as the heart does. We really can run (or walk, or bike, or swim) away from our problems—the everyday ones that cause pressure, tension, and anxiety to knot up our insides and put us in black moods.

Eileen Waters was one of the first American women ever to finish a 50-mile run. Several years earlier, her younger sister had committed suicide.

Eileen herself was understandably despondent over this family tragedy. To compensate, she ate compulsively. She started running to lose the weight she'd gained. She found that she lost her despair as well.

"Running just keeps me going," says Waters, "gets me out of my bad moods. It makes me feel good to be alive. I want to reach out to the world now, to touch it. I'm smiling a lot now."

Movement is strong medicine. Two researchers from the University of Southern California reported that a simple 15-minute walk was more relaxing than a tranquilizer drug.

Drs. Herbert de Vries and Gene Adams studied ten patients, ages 52 to 70. All showed above-average anxiety and tension levels. During one test, the patients took the tranquilizer in the prescribed dosage. Another day, they took a walk vigorous enough to raise their heart rate above 100 beats per minute. The walk had a greater calming effect, as measured by reduction of muscle tension and resting heart rate. Just 15 minutes of exercise soothed the patients for an hour after they'd stopped walking. And there were no harmful side effects.

The calming qualities of movement are rooted in heredity. Our ancestors reacted to threats in one of two ways: by preparing to stand their ground and fight, or preparing to flee the danger. Either way, the hormones readied the body for life-saving action.

Humans still face threats. In a crowded, fast-paced world, these are more subtle but just as real as those of our ancestors. But instead of following our instincts and fighting or fleeing, we go home and have a martini—or worse.

Our hormones have prepared us for action. If there isn't any, the tensions and anxieties, the urges to fight or flee, stay bottled up inside. Drugs treat the symptoms but not the causes.

Since modern life offers so much in the way of mental stress and so little in the way of release, we have to work hard at relaxing. Aerobic activity is one way.

This sounds contradictory—tensing the muscles to reduce tension. Yet a number of physiological investigations have shown that relaxation is most pronounced after heavy muscular work. Drs. Paul Insel and Walton Roth of Stanford University observe that "the most profound muscular and mental relaxation cannot be achieved by just trying to relax. The deepest relaxation, as measured by electrodes inserted in the muscles, follows a period of voluntarily increased muscular tension."

While the body works, the knot inside loosens. Exercise taken in proper doses is good and healthy mental medicine. It offers one of the few chances left to get our feet back on the ground, for the sake of our head.

"Chronic tension states," says Dr. Roth, "are known to be associated with numerous bodily malfunctions such as ulcers, migraine headaches, asthma, skin eruptions, high blood pressure, and even heart disease."

The symptoms on the psychological side are no prettier: "Irritability, touchiness, moodiness, and depression." These researchers add that aerobic exercise, notably running, "has been shown to relieve some of these symptoms."

Physical activity does this by pulling the plug on pent-up tension. The feeling of relief is familiar to anyone who runs. After most sessions, there is a feeling of relaxation—and sometimes even euphoria. Dr. Roth, a Stanford psychiatrist, noted these results in runners. "Of the group of thirty regular exercise participants," he says, "about three-quarters described a feeling of increased well-being that follows exercising. Often this was described as relief from tension or a feeling of calmness." Roth adds, "Probably the fact that the majority had sedentary occupations enhanced the effect of exercise. The extreme lack of physical activity during the working day seemed to result in a restlessness and tension."

He gives specifics in two cases. "One person felt no need for his scotch and water if he had exercised in the afternoon. Another claimed that he was able to think more clearly and felt less tired than when he missed his exercise."

Roth also has observed long-term psychological benefits from exercise. They match those identified by researchers Drs. A. H. Ismail and L. E. Trachtmann, who studied the effects of physical training on a group of previously inactive Purdue University faculty members.

"We were fairly sure," say Ismail and Trachtmann, "that our paunchy, sedentary, middle-aged academics were undergoing personality changes, subtly but definitely. By the time they reached the end of the [conditioning] program, they seemed to be interacting more freely and to be more relaxed. Their whole demeanor seemed to use to be more even, stable, and self-confident.

Ismail and Trachtmann checked their "off-the-cuff impressions," using scientific physiological and psychological testing methods. At the beginning of the four-month training period, some of these men could run no more than a quarter-mile. By the end of the study period, they were averaging 2 to 3 miles a day.

Among other testing, the researchers measured personality changes. They compared beginning exercisers with a high-fitness group, checking both groups before and after the training period on differences in four traits: emotional stability, imagination, self-sufficiency, and lack of guilt feelings.

The high-fitness group began with a healthier emotional profile (as measured by a standard psychological questionnaire) on all counts and scored consistently well after the four-month period. Imagination was these men's strongest point.

The low-fitness group's psychological ratings soared along with their physical condition in three of the four traits. For instance, they ended with an even higher self-sufficiency score than their already fit counterparts. Emotional stability "increased so markedly that there no longer was a significant difference between the groups," according to Drs. Ishmail and Trachtmann.

However, one result puzzled them. They thought guilt-proneness would drop as fitness increased. They say, "Persons with very high scores on [this factor] tend to be worried, anxious, depressed, easily overcome by moods, prone to depressions." This score should be low, as it was with men in the control group. It wasn't. It actually *increased* during the training period.

Ismail and Trachtmann explain that this may have been a temporary effect as the beginners realized the extent of their unfitness for the first time. They then felt guilty about not being able to get in shape immediately.

At any rate, the scores for the regular exercisers show what newcomers can expect once they have settled into their more active life.

Thought for the Day: Has your psychological outlook changed since you started exercising?

LESSON 42
The Pressure

Task for the Day: See the relationship between emotional stress and physical illness or injury.

Arthur Lydiard, the world's most honored running coach, had rarely been injured or ill in his more than sixty years. Suddenly, he was both at once. While recovering from knee surgery, he came down with a severe case of the flu. The two physical ailments probably weren't coincidental. The stress of his operation may have lowered his defenses against the virus.

A growing number of physicians believe that we don't catch diseases like the flu and colds; they *catch us.* These "bugs" attack constantly, but only gain a foothold when excessive stress pokes holes in our natural immunity.

The connection between stress and illness is strong. The same may be true for injuries. A researcher at Chico State University in California offers the theory that stresses apparently unrelated to physical training may lead to physical breakdowns during activity.

Dr. Walt Schafer thinks emotional traumas leave an exerciser more exposed to injury. He writes in his book *Stress, Distress and Growth* (International Dialogue Press, 1983), "Drs. Thomas H. Holmes and Richard H. Rahe developed a scale for measuring stresses associated with life events. On the basis of their research with thousands of people from all walks of life, they report that a person scoring less than 150 on this scale has only a 37 percent chance of becoming ill during the next two years. A score of 150 to 300 raises the odds of illness to 51 percent, and a 300-plus score means you have an 80 percent chance of becoming seriously ill."

The stressful life events listed in Table 11.1 range from death of a spouse (100 points) and divorce (73), down to a minor violation of the law (11 points). Dr. Schafer has evidence to show that the effects are felt as injuries as well as illnesses.

To test this theory, he studied questionnaires from nearly 600 runners. Schafer reports three key findings:

1. "The higher the life-change score for the past year," he says, "the greater number of running injuries during the past three months, the

Table 11.1
Stress Scores

Add up your emotional stresses from the past twelve months from this list compiled by Drs. Thomas H. Holmes and Richard H. Rahe. The higher your total score, the greater your statistical chances of suffering an illness or injury in the near future.

Event	Impact	Check for Yes
Death of spouse	100	_____
Divorce	73	_____
Marital separation	65	_____
Jail term	63	_____
Death of close family member	63	_____
Personal injury or illness	53	_____
Marriage	50	_____
Fired at work	47	_____
Marital reconciliation	45	_____
Retirement	45	_____
Change in health of family member	44	_____
Pregnancy	40	_____
Sex difficulties	39	_____
Gain of new family member	39	_____
Business readjustment	39	_____
Change in financial state	38	_____
Death of close friend	37	_____
Change to different line of work	36	_____
Change in arguments with spouse	35	_____
Mortgage over $10,000	31	_____
Foreclosure of mortgage or loan	30	_____
Change in responsibilities at work	29	_____
Son or daughter leaving home	29	_____
Trouble with in-laws	29	_____
Outstanding personal achievement	28	_____
Spouse begins or stops work	26	_____
Begin or end school	26	_____
Change in living conditions	25	_____
Revision of personal habits	24	_____
Trouble with boss	23	_____
Change in work hours or conditions	20	_____
Change in residence	20	_____
Change in schools	20	_____

Table 11.1—Continued

Event	Impact	Check for Yes
Change in recreation	19	_____
Change in church activities	19	_____
Change in social activities	18	_____
Mortgage or loan less than $10,000	17	_____
Change in sleeping habits	16	_____
Change in number of family gatherings	15	_____
Change in eating habits	15	_____
Vacation	13	_____
Christmas	12	_____
Minor violations of the law	11	_____

Your current total stress score: _____

more days of running missed during the past three months due to running injuries, and the more days of running reduced during the past three months due to running injuries."

2. The results were the same when Dr. Schafer examined the question, "Does the risk of running injuries increase when runners, for whatever reason, experience higher-than-usual personal stress during the past three months?"

3. He also found a direct link between injuries and chronic "Type-A behavior," which he defines as "a pattern of time urgency, intense drive to succeed, impatience, and hostility."

The conclusion: Whenever overall stress levels climb dangerously, try to lower those stressors over which you have control. Physical activity is one of those.

Schafer suggests, "Keep training during periods of high stress, but with moderation and sensitivity to early warning signs of injury and illness [see Week 5]. Back off in speed and distance when needed."

Think of yourself as a cup. Your capacity to accept the stresses of exercising is fixed. At any one time, you can only take so much work. If you try to pour in more than that amount, the excess spills over the top. At best, you gain nothing. At worst, you flood out your ability to do further work.

Many exercisers are latent workaholics who are attracted to aerobic activity because it seems to give free rein to that tendency. The harder they work, the more they think they can accomplish. But that isn't how it works when the cup runs over.

A man we'll simply call Don learned that the hard way. The lifelong athlete and professional fitness instructor had for years preached the need for leading a balanced life. Yet he now says, "I feel like a minister who suddenly realizes his son is a juvenile delinquent." He explains, "I almost made thirty years of running without any serious problems. But after turning 40, I became more competitive in my running and won numerous age-group events. I collected more trophies and medals in the next few years than in my previous twenty-five. My ego was on a continuous high. However. . ."

However, Don fell into a familiar trap. The more he won, the more he wanted to win—and the harder he worked at it. He also absorbed new job-related stresses. He exceeded his capacity to shoulder these burdens. His attitude was, "If I plan my work well and stay in top physical condition, nothing can bother me."

Wrong. He says that "in a period of approximately twelve months, all sorts of tensions hit me. I didn't realize the full impact until the end of the year. In December, I came down with my first serious injury and was on the verge of a nervous breakdown. I developed numerous symptoms and spent many hours in doctors' offices trying to discover what was wrong."

Here he defends his running. He says his "excellent physical condition was the only thing that prevented me from having a complete breakdown."

Only later did Don realize "what I had done to myself. I am now practicing a series of relaxation techniques on a daily basis. I am running with the fitness joggers [instead of training with other athletes]. I am sleeping 9 or 10 hours per night. I am not going to run any marathons in the foreseeable future, and all other races will be done at 80 percent effort."

On the job, this recovering workaholic says he has "delegated some responsibility to other staff members. I work normal hours, never taking anything home to work on in the evening." He adds that he has "learned that when the floodgates open, one should temper those stressors which are controllable. The others will drive you bananas if you don't. It is the total, cumulative effect that is dangerous."

Thought for the Day: *How would you lighten up if your physical and psychological stress load became too heavy to bear?*

LESSON 43
The Effort

Task for the Day: *Learn the value of doing less than your best.*

"Winning is easy," begins the actor in a television commercial. He's pretending to be ending a workout. He slam-dunks a basketball into a garbage can, then tears off his sweaty T-shirt in one motion. "Give 110 percent, expect 110 percent—from everyone, everything."

He's selling deodorant, and at the same time promoting one of the worst sports/fitness myths. All you have to do to win in sports and in life, the ad implies, is give more than your best. Look more closely at those lines. They're both contradictory and illogical. The terms *easy* and *110 percent* cancel each other out, and an effort beyond maximum is more than anyone can ever make.

Yet the myth dies hard. Athletes and exercisers think anything is possible if only they try harder. They run into more trouble from trying too hard than from doing too little. Overtrying is the greatest threat to the health and performance of an active person. Aerobic exercises put a premium on endurance and pacing, not on explosions of speed and power. Endurance activities demand that we ration our efforts and emotions over long distances, and penalize us for squandering all of our limited sources and leaving nothing for later. At any one time, then, we must intentionally do *less* than our best.

Trying to give 110 percent in training invites destruction. Working too hard, too often is the major cause of injury. At special risk are exercisers who take too little recovery time between hard efforts.

All-out work, challenging and exciting as it might be, tears us down. We repair that damage and prepare to accept more of it by staying well below the farthest distance and fastest pace we can manage. The best building seems to be done at about three-quarters effort.

You probably accept all this training advice with your head, even if your heart and legs don't always get the message. This book has drummed it into you almost from page one. What you may find harder to believe is that you can work better at your *maximum* by not trying to exceed it.

This has happened even with the world's fastest sprinters. Lee Evans still holds the world 400-meter dash record, set at the 1968 Olympics. Tommie Smith and John Carlos won 200-meter medals at the same Games. All were coached by the late Bud Winter.

Winter preached relaxation. "The way to run faster is with a four-fifths effort," Winter taught his runners. "Just take it nice and easy. Going all-out is counterproductive."

He might have exaggerated by calling for 80 percent effort. He told athletes this to restrain them from trying to give 110 percent and tying themselves in physical and emotional knots. An athlete or an exerciser is more likely to succeed by relaxing and letting the trained-in abilities flow out than by struggling and straining to exceed himself or herself.

"The key," said Winter, who was a former instructor of World War II pilots who had frozen at the controls when they tried too hard, "is learning to relax under the pressure of combat. Anyone who wants to do or die is as good as dead."

An even better word than relaxation might be *concentration*. Being relaxed implies not caring, not trying hard enough. Concentration means paying just enough attention to exactly what counts.

"Don't confuse concentration with consternation," warns sports psychologist Scott Pengelly. Consternation comes from focusing too strongly on a goal and trying too hard to make it come true. Concentration means tuning in to the signals coming from your own body and mind at that moment, tuning out distractions and letting what happens happen.

Thought for the Day: How well do you pace your efforts in physical training and in everyday life?

LESSON 44
The Pace

Task for the Day: Identify Type-A personality traits and their place in the race against time.

Twice each day, longtime exerciser Catherine runs or walks her two dogs. Well, the truth is that the big Lab drags her, and the little mongrel tries to do the same. They are impatient animals. No matter how fast their owner goes, it's always a step too slow for them.

The dogs strain against their leashes. If Catherine yanks them back, they pull all the harder to get away. All they do is tire themselves out and strain their necks, spoiling what could have been a pleasant outing if they had trotted along at the woman's side with some slack in their ropes.

"I know how they feel," says Catherine. "By nature, I'm like them. I strain against an invisible leash much of the day. No matter how fast it lets me go, I want to go a little faster. This wears me out and spoils many a pleasant outing."

She has conquered this tendency when she trains, and is working on it the rest of the day. She's trying to cure herself of the disease that is a national epidemic.

Dr. Meyer Friedman of San Francisco named it "hurry sickness." It starts from what he calls a "Type-A personality." He defines a Type-A person with masculine pronouns, but the symptoms apply equally to both sexes.

"He worries about the fact that he is dreadfully behind in doing all the things he should and could do," says Dr. Friedman. "Or he frets at delays in being seated in restaurants, boarding airplanes, being held up in traffic, and having people 'come to the point.' Or he frantically strives to obtain things worth *having* (a lovely home, a better position, a college education for his children) at the expense of the things worth *being* (a lover of the arts, a reader of good literature, and a devotee of the wonders of nature and mankind)."

Friedman is a heart specialist, and he worries about the Type-A person from that standpoint. "We're dead certain," he says, "that this personality is extraordinarily prone to coronary disease. What I am saying—and we have much data to support it—is that whenever a man struggles too incessantly to accomplish too many things in too little space of time (thus engendering a sense of time urgency), or whenever a man struggles too competitively with other individuals, this struggle markedly accentuates the course of coronary disease."

Even if physical symptoms never surface, hurry sickness still makes life a rather miserable grind. Physical activity can contribute to the problem or be part of the cure, depending on how it is paced.

Ambition has its place. We sometimes have to reach beyond what we are, toward what we might become. We sometimes have to rush and strain to get there. But we can't work that way all the time. Much of what we call "being ambitious" is nothing more than tugging against a leash that won't yield. No matter how fast it lets us go, we want to go faster. We gain nothing from this struggle except fatigue and pain.

Thought for the Day: *Can you think of a better way to win the race against time than to drop out?*

Now turn to Table 11.2 to log in your training time for the week.

Table 11.2
Week 11 Training Chart

Record your physical training for the week, including only formal sessions, not incidental daily exercise. List the actual date, aerobic activity, duration in minutes, and any supplemental "muscle" exercises. A suggested weekly program would include four aerobic training days, lasting at least 30 minutes, with not more than two training days in a row or more than two straight rest days.

Day (Date)	Aerobic Exercise	Duration	Other Exercise
Sunday			
Monday			
Tuesday			
Wednesday			
Thursday			
Friday			
Saturday			

Total aerobic training time for the week: _____

Number of aerobic sessions: _____

Average time per session: _____

WEEK 12

Self-Improvement

LESSON 45
The Bonuses

Task for the Day: Recognize benefits besides physical ones that come with the aerobic activity package.

"*The loneliness of the long-distance runner*": This phrase has endured as a cliche ever since Allan Sillitoe wrote a short novel and later a screenplay by that title in the 1960s. The story was fiction, and so is the usual usage of the word *lonely* as it applies to runners and similar athletes and exercisers. Don't feel sorry for the lone active person. This apparent loneliness is neither a negative factor nor a necessary evil of the activity. Many people *prefer* to train by themselves. It may be the only chance they get to escape crowds. The solitude is self-sought. This is a quiet time for contemplation.

On the other hand, an exerciser who wants this to be a sociable activity can plug into a support system. Training with a partner or a small group inspires conversation. Traveling together for long periods of time, with no other entertainment at hand, breaks down barriers to communication.

Dr. Thaddeus Kostrubala was among the first psychiatrists to use running as a therapeutic tool. He says patients bare their souls more completely after at least a 30-minute run than at any other time. Dr. Kostrubala says his patients often feel terrible early in their runs. But if he nurses them through these doldrums and keeps them moving for 30 minutes or more, their symptoms improve. The most productive therapy sessions follow this amount of training.

Longtime runners will tell you only half-jokingly that running develops one set of muscles more thoroughly than any other: those that operate the mouth. Those same muscles are also the last to tire.

The compulsion to talk about aerobic activity is nearly matched by the urge to write about it. Many exercisers keep diaries that preserve their statistics and experiences in loving detail. More than a few of these writers make their observations public in magazines and books.

Dozens of national magazines cover fitness activities generally or individual sports specifically. Hundreds of books have been published in this field, with new ones appearing every month.

Besides all that it does for you physically, aerobic activity encourages thinking and talking. It inspires you to write out your thoughts and read those of people like yourself. This benefits package costs very little and repays you with interest.

Thought for the Day: *Do you spend time exercising, or do you invest it profitably?*

LESSON 46
The Thinking

Task for the Day: *Reserve time to be by yourself and to think about yourself.*

The nature of endurance activities often makes the exerciser a loner by necessity. You might consider becoming one by choice.

Learn to enjoy your own company. Cultivate aloneness as one of the hidden rewards of training instead of constantly seeking out partners as if this were a tennis match. Take advantage of this rare chance to get away from people and the talk they generate. All day long, you're subjected to talk—out loud and on paper, live and recorded. You wake up in the morning to the news talk on the clock radio. You eat breakfast to the talk in the newspaper or on the back of the cereal box. The day's work is a series of talking in meetings, sales negotiations, business luncheons, letters, and reports. At school you absorb lectures, answer tests questions, and write papers. You drive your car to the talk of DJs on the radio, the singers on the tape deck, or the trucker on the CB. You talk to your family or friends over dinner, and the TV talks to you until bedtime.

Only one kind of talking is missing from this day. You haven't left time to talk with yourself. You haven't allowed a quiet, uninterrupted time in which to mull over your own ideas.

Call timeout. Set aside one hour in twenty-four that is yours alone. Guard it jealously against all intruders—human, print, or electronic. In all of your other waking hours, your head is being cluttered with the information, opinions, orders, and demands of others. Keep this one hour as your time to remove that clutter and replace it with clarity of thought.

Give yourself the full hour, even if it is only partially filled with physical training on some days and contains none at all on others. Get away from chaos for that hour. Separate yourself from all that is crowded, noisy, and distracting.

The beauty of exercising alone is that you can't take the external voices with you. (Not, that is, unless you wear a stereo headset—a high-tech way to spoil this natural beauty.) You move away for a little while from TV and radio, from newspapers and books, from employees and bosses, from teachers and students.

You then get that essential time to be alone, to clear away cluttered thoughts, to reflect, to plan, to dream.

A stock question asked by people who don't exercise aerobically of those who do is, "What do you think about all that time you're out there training by yourself?"

The best answer would be, "Nothing much."

We can't, of course, completely stop thinking any more than we can quit breathing. But we can stop worrying about serious matters, and instead let the mind float or leap from subject to subject. Relax the mind, in other words. Meditate on the move.

People who would never call what they do "meditation" still practice it regularly. This head-clearing happens almost automatically when a few basic conditions are met.

Dr. William Glasser lists them as part of his theory of positive addiction, which differs from the negative type in that it builds mental and physical strength instead of sapping it. This psychiatrist's research shows that aerobic exercisers tend to become positively addicted to their activity. The chance to meditate is one of the attractions.

Dr. Glasser gives several hints for promoting both the addictive and meditative qualities of aerobic exercise:

1. *Train alone* when you want to clear your thoughts. A second voice doesn't let you hear your own clearly enough.
2. *Simplify.* Train on a safe, uncomplicated route and by a simple routine that doesn't demand constant attention.
3. *Go gently.* Train at a steady, comfortable pace. If you're too tired, all you can think about is how much you hurt and when you get to stop hurting.
4. *Allow time.* Give yourself a 30-minute minimum. It may take that long just to clear away the mental clutter.
5. *Daydream.* Put your physical activity on automatic pilot, and let your mind roam wherever it wants to go.

"I have talked with many addicted [exercisers], runners, and others," says Dr. Glasser, "and it is this state of mind that almost all of them describe: a trance-like, transcendental mental state that accompanies the addictive exercise."

Forget those fancy words. You are essentially doing garbage processing. The brain acts as a trash bin, collecting sensory stimuli at an astounding rate. You're usually so busy taking in sights, sounds, and smells that you don't have time to process them all. Escaping from overstimulation, into exercise in this case, gives you a chance to catch up. You can stand aside and watch ideas float past as if they're pieces of garbage of a conveyor belt. You can poke casually through the information, plucking out the few bits worth recycling, and letting the waste fall away.

You should feel good afterward, both for the few meaningful thoughts you saved and the many meaningless ones you discarded.

Thought for the Day: What do you think about while training?

LESSON 47
The Talking

Task for the Day: See the practical and social values of teaming up.

You were just advised getting away from people during training. Now you're urged to get together with them then. Confused? Don't be. This can be either a time to think or to talk. Contemplation and conversation can at different times each play a role in your exercise routine, as they do for Dr. George Sheehan.

Dr. Sheehan often plans much of his writing on the run. "I take the raw material out onto the road with me," he says, "with the hope that during the run the one sentence that will set up the entire organization of the column will somehow come to me. More often than not, it does. But I can't force it. I have to wait for it to come."

Other voices would block those thoughts. Yet Sheehan doesn't always go out to think. Sometimes he welcomes talk.

"Running frees me from the monosyllabic inanities of my usual tongue-tied state," he says. "It liberates me from the polysyllabic jargon of my profession. It removes me from the kind of talk that aims at concealing rather than revealing what is in my heart." He adds that "for me, no time passes faster than when running with a companion. An hour of conversation on the run is one of the quickest and most satisfying hours ever spent."

Just as you might have started exercising alone because you had no choice—and now continue that way because you learned to like being by yourself—you may team up for practical reasons and keep coming back for social ones. The practical reason is mutual support. You can train farther and easier as a team or group than you would alone. Just as exercising alone opens up time you might otherwise never take for traveling with yourself, training with others gives you time for talking that you might not otherwise do.

Something about aerobic activity encourages conversation, just as it coaxes out thought. Perhaps the rhythm of striding, pedaling, or stroking over long periods jars loose ideas that otherwise might be held inside. Maybe even dressing the same symbolically strips us of the roles we carry the rest of the day and frees us from the verbal posturing we do then.

More likely, the talk flows freely because people who enjoy each other's company are sharing an interest and effort. The activity period gives them uninterrupted time to converse. Here are a few hints for forming a training group and keeping it harmonious:

1. *Make it rewarding.* Offer something in the group effort (besides the talk) that an exerciser can't or won't find alone. For instance, a weekly extra-long training session at a special location.
2. *Keep it small.* Two is the minimum number, of course, but leaves no spares if someone is absent. More than five makes the group unwieldy and impersonal. Three or four is an ideal group size.
3. *Think and act alike.* Form a group with similar abilities and ambitions. Nothing splits you up faster than disagreements over paces and distances.
4. *Be regular.* Have a regular, agreed-upon meeting place and time so no one has to make special scheduling arrangements.
5. *Stay together.* Train at the pace of the slowest person so you can all get in on the conversation.

Thought for the Day: Do you have a friend or family member with whom you want to train and talk?

LESSON 48
The Writing

Task for the Day: Read what others have written about fitness, and write down your experiences with it.

YOUR READING

This book's author drew upon many sources for information and inspiration. If you want to learn more about subjects introduced here, go to some of those sources yourself. Here's an alphabetical list of selected authors who gave the most help:

Covert Bailey writes about the connection between exercise and weight control in his book *Fit or Fat?* (Houghton Mifflin, 1977).

Dr. Kenneth Cooper laid the groundwork for all the fitness writers who followed. His books, all published originally by M. Evans and Company, include *Aerobics,* 1968; *The Aerobics Program for Total Health and Well-Being,* 1982; *The New Aerobics,* 1970; and *Running without Fear,* 1985.

Dr. David Costill, an exercise physiologist, studies the body's reactions to training. He reports many of them in *A Scientific Approach to Distance Running* (Tafnews Press, 1978).

Dr. Herbert de Vries discusses the science of activity in *Physiology of Exercise for Physical Education and Athletics* (William C. Brown, 1986).

Joe Henderson, this book's author, has many other titles to his credit: *Jog Run Race* (1977), *The Long Run Solution* (1976), *Run Farther Run Faster* (1979) and *Run Gently Run Long* (1974), all from Anderson/World; *Running for Fitness for Sport and for Life* (1985), *Running Handbook* (1986) and *Running Your Best Race* (1985), all from William C. Brown; and *Running, A to Z* (Stephen Greene Press, 1983).

Ian Jackson combines the philosophies and practices of yoga and aerobic exercise in *The Breathplay Approach to Whole Life Fitness* (Doubleday, 1986), and *New Exercises for Runners* and *Yoga and the Athlete* (Anderson/World, 1978).

Arthur Lydiard, a coach of New Zealand Olympic champions, promotes healthy aerobic activity in *Running for Your Life* (Minerva, 1965), and *Running the Lydiard Way* (Anderson/World, 1978).

Tom Osler balances the wish for short-term performance gains and the need to maintain long-term health in his *Serious Runner's Handbook* (Anderson/World, 1978).

Dr. Walt Schafer discusses the connection of exercise and stress in *Stress Management for Wellness* (Holt, Rinehart and Winston, 1987).

Dr. George Sheehan, whose theories and practices support this book, has written several of his own: *Dr. Sheehan on Fitness* (1983), *Running and Being* (1978) and *This Running Life* (1980), all from Simon and Schuster; *Dr. Sheehan on Running* (1975), *Encyclopedia of Athletic Medicine* (1972) and *Medical Advice for Runners* (1978), all from Anderson/World.

Dr. Steven Subtonick, a podiatrist, authored *Cures for Common Running Injuries* in 1979 and *The Running Foot Doctor* in 1977, both for Anderson/World.

Dr. Peter Wood, a researcher on the medical benefits of exercise, wrote *The California Diet and Exercise Program* (Anderson/World, 1983) and *Run to Health* (Charter Books, 1980).

YOUR BOOK

Someone else's writing can only put you on the starting line. From there, you must go your own way, then tell what you did there in your own words and numbers (as this book has encouraged you to do with its weekly logs, such as Table 12.1). A diary helps give your life stories happier endings.

You can be your own biographer. You don't have to be a talented writer to profit from a diary. You don't have to spend more than a minute a day writing in it. You don't even have to write many, if any, words. Numbers alone tell stories as they recall old training sessions and suggest new possibilities.

That process begins with three guidelines:

1. *Keep it simple.* Limit the amount of information to a few essentials that can be listed briefly, quickly, and in accessible form for review. The harder it is to keep a diary, the less likely you are to use it.

   You don't need a preprinted training diary. A calendar with large blocks of space will do nicely as long as it is tacked to your bedroom or office wall, but it won't travel or store well. A notebook works best for this purpose. Fill it at the rate of one or two or a few lines a day.

2. *Keep it up.* Analyze the accumulating data over extended periods of time to judge your results. Review at the end of each week, month, and year. The longer you maintain the diary, the clearer become your patterns of response to the exercise—and the clearer your thinking about it.

   Days of training leave behind what appear to be random footsteps in the diary. You can't take much direction from them at first. But the weeks, months, and years form a trail that points two ways. It shows where you have been and where you might go next.

3. *Keep it.* Store your records in a safe place, treating them as the precious volumes they will become in time. Their value grows along with their age and bulk.

   The ultimate value of a diary is as a personal library of memories and dreams. You can open it to any old page and bring a day back to life. You can call up a mental videotape and, from a few statistics on the page, recreate all you did and felt that day.

These recordings give substance and permanence to efforts that otherwise would be as temporary as the moment and to experiences that would be as invisible as footprints on the pavement.

Thought for the Day: *Did you record your training and thoughts today?*

Now turn to Table 12.1 to log in your training time for the week.

Table 12.1
Week 12 Training Chart

Record your physical training for the week, including only formal sessions, not incidental daily exercise. List the actual date, aerobic activity, duration in minutes, and any supplemental "muscle" exercises. A suggested weekly program would include four aerobic training days, lasting at least 30 minutes, with not more than two training days in a row or more than two straight rest days.

Day (Date)	Aerobic Exercise	Duration	Other Exercise
Sunday			
Monday			
Tuesday			
Wednesday			
Thursday			
Friday			
Saturday			

Total aerobic training time for the week: _____

Number of aerobic sessions: _____

Average time per session: _____

WEEK 13

Self-Preservation

LESSON 49
The Warranty

> ***Task for the Day:*** *Review the practices that delay the physical effects of aging.*

"We are born," says Dr. George Sheehan, "with a seventy-year warranty. Three score and ten, the Bible promises us. But many Americans will never see it, because they never bother to read the instructions."

Never mind that our biologically programmed lifespan, as identified by scientists, is now significantly higher than seventy years. We won't argue here with Biblical wisdom and the point Dr. Sheehan is making.

Study the warranty, he advises. "The instructions when we left Eden were simple enough: a six-day work week, and work that would bring sweat to our brow."

That type of work isn't required of most people any more. That doesn't make it any less important. Sheehan says that "the sweat of our brow, no longer necessary to earn our daily bread, has become even more necessary to make us fully functioning men and women. It now determines whether or not we will live a full seventy years, and live them at our full physical potential." He adds, "Humans do not have a built-in obsolescence. We are not made to break down, rust out, or come apart at an early age."

Humans break down because of owner abuse and neglect, which the standard warranty doesn't cover. Upkeep is the owner's responsibility. That involves proper use and the right kind of fuel. Proper use means physical activity, particularly aerobic. Fuel means food of the right type and amount.

The collapse starts from the inside—with heart and lungs that grow flabby, with blood vessels that get clogged, with a blanket of fat under the skin. The repair starts by reversing those conditions.

Aerobic activity, combined with a sensible diet, can train the cardiovascular system, flush out the plumbing and eat away the fat. All of this helps keep the body young for its years.

Dr. Michael Pollock tested endurance athletes aged 40 and older. "It was particularly interesting to note the high maximum oxygen uptake results," says Pollock of this reading for aerobic capacity. These athletes used oxygen as effectively as the untrained typical person half their age. He adds, "Resting heart rate and body fat were much lower in the tested runners than in the sedentary population." Pulse rates were 10 to 20 beats per minute below average for their age group. Body fat was about half the expected percentage.

However, cholesterol readings were below average only in athletes who watched what they ate. Dr. Pollock says, "This agrees with other research findings that serum cholesterol appears to be affected more by diet than by exercise."

"Too little exercise plus too much saturated fat, sugar, and salt cancel out the warranty," says Dr. George Sheehan. The result is an epidemic of early breaking down, rusting out, and coming apart.

Can anything be done about this? Of course. Go back to the original instructions, work up a daily sweat, eat naturally, and the breakdown can be fixed or prevented.

Thought for the Day: *Are you living up to the conditions of your lifetime warranty?*

LESSON 50
The Age

Task for the Day: *Adopt a positive attitude toward aging.*

Satchel Paige pitched major-league baseball when his age was somewhere between the late 40s and early 60s. He either wasn't sure how old he was or wasn't telling.

Paige coined homespun philosophies that outlived his playing career. He's known best as the man who warned us not to look back, because someone might be gaining on us.

Once, when asked the inevitable question about his age, Paige answered with a question of his own: "How old would you be if you didn't know how old you were?" Think about that. If you didn't know the year you were born, how old would you judge yourself to be? There is no more accurate test of true age than that. You can't tell by looking at your teeth, as we would with a horse, or by sawing yourself in half and counting rings, as with a tree. You literally are as old as you feel.

Shirali Mislimov was the world's oldest man when he died at a reputed 168. The Soviet citizen had said, "There are two sources of long life. One is a gift of nature—the pure air and clean water of the mountains [where he lived], the fruit of the earth, peace, rest, the soft and warm climate of the highlands. The second source is people. He lives long who enjoys life and who bears no jealousy of others, whose heart harbors no malice or anger, who sings a lot and cries a little, who rises and retires with the sun, who likes to work and knows how to rest."

Some of the world's longest living people reside in the Pakistani territory of Hunza. That kingdom's ruler once stated, "The keynote of life is growth, not aging. The life that flows through us at 80 is the same that energized us in infancy. It does not get old or weak. So-called age is the deterioration of enthusiasm, faith to live, and will to progress."

Larry Lewis of San Francisco ran and walked and worked as a waiter until a few months before his death at 106. He always hated the word *old.* "Never say a person is so many years *old,*" Lewis once snapped at a reporter. "Old means dilapidated and something you eventually get rid of, like an old automobile or refrigerator. You're like a violin, a portrait, a wine. You mellow, but you never grow old."

Aging is not a death warrant. It's an opportunity to grow, to keep moving, to keep enjoying. Aging has a plus side. With it comes the following benefits:

- The pride of still performing well, even though you have put on more than a few miles.

- The wisdom that comes with experience, and the experience to use wisely what you know.

- The patience to let things happen at their own pace rather than trying to make them happen quickly.

- The confidence to go your own way, in your own way, at your own pace— without worrying about how other people do things or expect you to do them.

- The hardness that comes with absorbing decades of knocks, and the softness that comes with adjusting to change instead of fighting it.

Thought for the Day: How old do you feel?

LESSON 51
The End

Task for the Day: Think about the inevitable.

Fitness doesn't guarantee immunity to life-threatening conditions. Neither does being a doctor. Dr. George Sheehan got his first hint of trouble to come while visiting another fitness pioneer, Dr. Kenneth Cooper, at the Aerobics Center in Dallas. Dr. Cooper couldn't pass up the chance to give Sheehan a complete physical exam.

Jim Fixx, the author of a best-selling running book, had declined Cooper's offer the year before. Fixx died shortly afterward of heart disease that might have been detected. Cooper wasn't going to let Sheehan slip through the net, too.

"That was when he discovered this suspicious area in my prostate," George said after his test, before he knew how serious his condition might be. "The news was paralyzing. I was suddenly aware of my mortality."

He had a growth biopsied, then sweated out a week of waiting to hear the results. "Whether this nodule turned out to be benign or malignant," he said at the time, "my life had been unalterably changed."

After hearing a good report then, Sheehan noted, "The week of waiting had led me to the truth. This was no pardon I had received. It was a temporary stay. Eventually, I would come to justice. I had been granted a little more time to deal with the inevitable."

He was given two more years before he had to face the inevitable even more directly than before. Then a second biopsy revealed he had an unstoppable cancer. After recovering from the initial shock, Dr. Sheehan resolved to keep running (as well as walking, biking, and swimming), writing, and speaking as long and as well as possible.

"In my lectures on fitness," he said then, "I have always put down the argument that it extends life. I ask who runs out of concern about longevity. I answer that question in the next breath: no one. What we are interested in is *performance*. Our consuming concern is getting up in the morning and doing our best the rest of the day." Thinking about that answer later, Sheehan added, "But what is performance but our best rebuttal to mortality. Daily, by deed or subterfuge, we make our argument against the essential truth of the human condition."

He said he didn't continue training "with the anticipation that it will do anything for my cancer. I run in order to remain as healthy as possible, regardless of what the disease does to me." Sheehan then switched to talking as a doctor would about someone's illness other than his own: "The patient does have some control over the impact that the disease has on his life. Mainly, in trying to live each day to the fullest potential he can exert that control. There is a healthy way to be ill."

George once said that after all he has done as a doctor, runner, writer, and speaker, he still thinks of himself as an "underachiever." "That's the main reason why I'm not sitting watching the ocean. I could do that. I've paid my dues. Lots of people my age [late 60s] are sitting in Florida now. But I feel I've never achieved what I could. I haven't run as well as I can, I haven't spoken as well as I can, and I haven't written as well as I can. If you take less than that view, you're finished."

Thought for the Day: *If fitness didn't add one day to your life-span, would you still work to gain and maintain it?*

LESSON 52
The Values

Task for the Day: *Look for measures of success and satisfaction in your fitness program.*

A sad result of running author Jim Fixx's death from a heart attack, suffered while running, is the impression left with the general public that he lived a lie and died in vain. Runners and other exercisers have been challenged with the question, "If this is so good for you, why didn't it save him?"

The best answer is that Fixx didn't train primarily to save his life or to extend it, nor do most of us. He may have started running out of fear for his health. But he soon discovered, as you probably have, that more positive benefits kept him going. Fixx knew, as you do, that training is less a physical act than a mental and emotional exercise. The physiological results are less immediate and dramatic than the psychological ones. Those can be found in other activities that provide a chance to be a winner, a way to be creative, a place to feel heroic. Fitness activity offers all three values at once.

WINNER

A winner never quits. So the way to keep yourself from stopping is to recognize true victories. This requires broader definitions of winning and losing than the athletic, fitness, and business worlds generally use. Consider these redefinitions:

- Winning is realizing you have already won by becoming active. You stand out from the masses who are content to let machines do their moving for them. Losing is promising to get into better shape on a tomorrow that never comes.

- Winning is finishing the distance you set for yourself, however long it might take. Speed is a gift, but endurance and persistence are earned. Losing is dropping out for no other reason than weak will.

- Winning is measuring yourself only against your own standards. It is realizing that the only person who can beat you is you. Losing is blaming your losses on anyone but yourself.

- Winning is working with other people so all of your results can be better than any of you could have achieved alone. Losing is interfering with someone else's chances to win.

- Winning is knowing you are only as good as your most recent effort. Fitness doesn't store well, so you must renew it regularly. Losing is living in the past. Losing has no future, while winning lasts.

ARTIST

Aerobic training gives you a rare chance to take complete charge of your own actions and thoughts. You alone choose the distance and pace. The efforts are all yours. So are the rewards.

For that hour, you take full command of and responsibility for what you do and think. It may be your quietest and calmest and most productive time all day. This is when you find out who you are and what you can do at an elemental level.

Much of life is defined by what we *have:* job, house, address, degrees, titles, clothes, cars. None of that counts when we train for aerobic fitness. We strip down to who we *are*—a body and mind facing the elements of time, distance, and environment.

The pleasures you get from a training session are both free and priceless. You can have them any day, but no amount of money can buy them. Only effort can.

You and the elements are like a painter's canvas and brush, a writer's paper and pen, or a sculptor's granite and chisel. These raw materials are nothing special until the artist decides to make something of them. Anyone has the materials at hand, but it takes special care to turn them into art.

One definition of art is an uncommon piece made from common materials. An artist is one who brings order and beauty to the random events of life, who sees common things in uncommon ways. By these definitions, you are an artist when you exercise. You made something from next to nothing. The abilities you now possess didn't exist a short while ago, and they would soon disappear if you left them unused.

You have created a monument to yourself. Now preserve it in this condition or continue the polishing.

HERO

Most people still have heroes instead of being one. They rank themselves by other people's standards and don't match up. They don't try for fear of failing. They never let themselves be proud of themselves.

This is a shame, because winning at the race of life isn't reserved for the people who cross the finish line first. Anyone who enters can win.

This doesn't mean that winning is automatic. If it were, victories wouldn't mean anything. There would be no challenge. But the odds of winning are in the player's favor.

In life, as in sport, the risk of defeat adds to the thrill of victory. Winning requires work—honest, intelligent effort. But in life, unlike in most sports, the number of potential winners is unlimited. You aren't required to beat anyone else to win, but only to match or exceed your own expectations.

This attitude starts in your aerobic exercise sessions, but it shouldn't stop there. Be your own hero there, and you can become one anywhere.

Thought for the Day: Are you a winner, artist and hero to yourself?

Now turn to Table 13.1 to log in your training time for the week.

Table 13.1
Week 13 Training Chart

Record your physical training for the week, including only formal sessions, not incidental daily exercise. List the actual date, aerobic activity, duration in minutes, and any supplemental "muscle" exercises. A suggested weekly program would include four aerobic training days, lasting at least 30 minutes, with not more than two training days in a row or more than two straight rest days.

Day (Date)	Aerobic Exercise	Duration	Other Exercise
Sunday			
Monday			
Tuesday			
Wednesday			
Thursday			
Friday			
Saturday			

Total aerobic training time for the week: _____

Number of aerobic sessions: _____

Average time per session: _____

Index